Pandemic Supplements

© Copyright: Steven Magee 2023

Edition 1

Cover Pictures: Steven Magee testing "Pandemic Supplements" at 36,000 feet in a pressurized airplane. His pulse oximeter is reading 91% SpO2, which is considered worrisome by the medical profession. The rear cover shows him researching at the Oregon State Hospital Museum of Mental Health:

https://oshmuseum.org/

Contents

5

Introduction

Pandemic Supplements came about after fifteen years of largely unsuccessful treatments from the medical profession. I had a wide variety of strange ailments that started my regular visits to doctors offices in 2006 at age thirty-six. Instead of getting healthier under the care of the medical profession, I became sicker!

I was so sick in my forties that I could not work and I was telling my family I expected to die before fifty! As it turned out, I was probably right. By my mid-forties I was heavily experimenting with nutritional supplements, looking for improved health.

In 2015 at age forty-five, I developed a serious flu-like illness that completely wrecked my mental and physical health! It was a nightmare. By 2016 I was on a CPAP machine and a few years later a BiPAP machine due to low blood oxygen levels during sleep. I was sicker than ever and constantly fatigued!

Using nutritional supplements and lifestyle changes I started to see health improvements in my late forties. Instead of being dead by fifty, I was slowly improving my health! That improvement has continued through to age fifty-three when I wrote this book.

I am sharing the fruits of my discoveries with you, so you can work with your doctor on improving your own health. I got smart and my smart techniques are in this book! At the time of writing, the COVID-19 pandemic was in its fourth year and long COVID was prevalent in the population. The nutritional supplements discussed in this book are being linked to improved health outcomes in both conditions.

I have an extensive history of cold and flu-like illnesses during my adult years. I started my career working in one of the largest teaching and university research hospitals in Europe and had flu-like illnesses there, I had been to South Korea during the influenza A/H1N1 pandemic (Swine Flu) and developed a flu-like illness there, I had regularly worked with international people and I had been exposed to the international university environment and had flu-like illnesses during that time.

A significant health collapse had occurred after contracting a severe flu-like illness from an international professor at the local university in 2015. I did not know it at the time, but the range of physical and mental health symptoms that developed in me afterward are now called "Long COVID"! That professor was never healthy afterwards and died two years later.

The three supplement protocols detailed in this book were developed during the COVID-19 pandemic. The long COVID symptoms I was displaying significantly subsided by using the three supplement protocols. I have much better mental and physical health today. I look better too!

This book contains the very latest research on health and the human environment. It should be viewed as the current ideas and the contents are subject to review by the medical community. The author and publisher accept no liability whatsoever for any of the contents and the book is published in the spirit of unrestricted access to the latest ideas and medical theories in a changing world. These are experimental health techniques and the long term side effects are unknown.

You should always consult with a licensed and certified medical professional on any aspects of health, sickness or disease.

"Smart people realize the smartest person that can fix their health issues is themselves!"

Steven Magee

Long COVID?

It was clear my flu-like sickness in 2015 had triggered a sickness that resembled "Long COVID". But long COVID was unknown in 2015, so how could I have had it? Coronavirus has been in global circulation since the 1960's. There are seven types and COVID-19 is just the latest one. There were six others that came before it!

The Wikipedia article *"Coronavirus"* states: *"Six species of human coronaviruses are known, with one species subdivided into two different strains, making seven strains of human coronaviruses altogether. Seasonal distribution of HCoV-NL63 in Germany shows a preferential detection from November to March. Four human coronaviruses produce symptoms that are generally mild, even though it is contended they might have been more aggressive in the past:*

- *Human coronavirus OC43 (HCoV-OC43), β-CoV.*

- *Human coronavirus HKU1 (HCoV-HKU1), β-CoV.*

- *Human coronavirus 229E (HCoV-229E), a-CoV.*

- *Human coronavirus NL63 (HCoV-NL63), a-CoV–.*

Three human coronaviruses produce potentially severe symptoms:

- *Severe acute respiratory syndrome coronavirus (SARS-CoV), β-CoV (identified in 2003).*

- *Middle East respiratory syndrome-related coronavirus (MERS-CoV), β-CoV (identified in 2012).*

- *Severe acute respiratory syndrome coronavirus 2 (SARS-CoV-2), β-CoV (identified in 2019).*

These cause the diseases commonly called SARS, MERS, and COVID-19 respectively."

https://en.wikipedia.org/wiki/Coronavirus

As you can see, it is possible for a person to have been infected with coronavirus since the 1960's! Regarding long COVID, The Wikipedia article *"Long COVID"* states:

"Long COVID is a condition characterized by long-term consequences persisting or appearing after the typical convalescence period of COVID-19. It is also known as post-COVID-19 syndrome, post-COVID-19 condition, post-acute sequelae of COVID-19 (PASC), or chronic COVID syndrome (CCS). Long COVID can affect nearly every organ system, with sequelae including respiratory system disorders, nervous system and neurocognitive disorders, mental health disorders, metabolic disorders, cardiovascular disorders, gastrointestinal disorders, musculoskeletal pain, and anemia. A wide range of symptoms are commonly reported, including fatigue, malaise, headaches, shortness of breath, anosmia (loss of smell), parosmia (distorted smell), muscle weakness, low fever and cognitive dysfunction.

The exact nature of symptoms and the number of people who experience long-term symptoms are unknown; these vary according to the definition used, the population being studied, and the time period used in the study. A survey by the UK Office for National Statistics estimated that about 14% of people who tested positive for SARS-CoV-2 experienced one or more symptoms for longer than three months. A study from the University of Oxford of 273,618 survivors of COVID-19, mainly from the United States, showed that about 37% experienced one or more symptoms between three and six months after diagnosis.

While studies into various aspects of long COVID are under way, as of November 2021, the definition of the illness is still unclear, as is its mechanism. Health systems in some countries and jurisdictions have been mobilized to deal with this group of patients by creating specialized clinics and providing advice. Overall, however, it is considered by default to be a diagnosis of exclusion.

A review suggests that global prevalence of long COVID conditions after infection could be as high as 43%, with the most common symptoms being fatigue and memory problems."

https://en.wikipedia.org/wiki/Long_COVID

The term "Long COVID" was first used in May 2020 and the disease is in the early stages of being defined. There are a number of international definitions. Wikipedia states:

"The World Health Organization (WHO) established a clinical case definition in October 2021, published in the journal The Lancet Infectious Diseases: post-COVID-19 condition occurs in individuals with a history of probable or confirmed SARS-CoV-2 infection, usually 3 months from the onset, with symptoms that last for at least 2 months and cannot be explained by an alternative diagnosis. Common symptoms include, but are not limited to, fatigue, shortness of breath, and cognitive dysfunction, and generally have an impact on everyday functioning. Symptoms might be new onset following initial recovery from an acute COVID-19 episode or persist from the initial illness. Symptoms might also fluctuate or relapse over time.

The British National Institute for Health and Care Excellence (NICE) divides COVID-19 into three clinical case definitions: acute COVID-19 for signs and symptoms during the first four weeks after infection with severe acute respiratory syndrome coronavirus 2 (SARS-CoV-2) is the first, and long Covid for new or ongoing symptoms four weeks or more after the start of acute COVID-19, which is divided into the other two: ongoing symptomatic COVID-19 for effects from four to twelve weeks after onset, and post-COVID-19 syndrome for effects that persist 12 or more weeks after onset. NICE describes the term long COVID, which it uses "in addition to the clinical case definitions", as "commonly used to describe signs and symptoms that continue or develop after acute COVID-19. It includes both ongoing symptomatic COVID-19 (from four to twelve weeks) and post-COVID-19 syndrome (12 weeks or more)". NICE defines post-COVID-19 syndrome as "Signs and symptoms that develop during or after an infection consistent with COVID-19, continue for more than 12 weeks and are not explained by an alternative diagnosis. It usually presents with clusters of symptoms, often overlapping, which can fluctuate and change over time and can affect any system in the body. Post-COVID-19 syndrome may be considered before 12 weeks while the possibility of an alternative underlying disease is also being assessed"

In February 2021, the U.S. National Institutes of Health (NIH) director Francis Collins indicated long COVID symptoms for individuals who "don't recover fully over a period of a few weeks" be collectively referred to as "Post-Acute Sequelae of SARS-CoV-2 Infection" (PASC). The NIH listed long COVID symptoms of fatigue, shortness of breath, brain fog, sleep disorders, intermittent fevers, gastrointestinal symptoms, anxiety, and depression. Symptoms can persist for months and can range from mild to incapacitating, with new symptoms arising well after the time of infection. The Centers for Disease Control and Prevention (CDC) term Post-Covid Conditions qualifies long Covid as symptoms four or more weeks after first infection."

https://en.wikipedia.org/wiki/Long_COVID

Long COVID has a wide range of symptoms associated with it and Wikipedia states:

"Symptoms reported by people with long COVID include:

- *Extreme fatigue.*

- *Long-lasting cough.*

- *Muscle weakness.*

- *Low grade fever.*

- *Inability to concentrate (brain fog).*

- *Memory lapses.*

- *Mental health problems, such as changes in mood or depression.*

- *Sleep difficulties.*

- *Headaches.*

- *Joint pain.*

- *Needle pains in arms and legs.*

- *Diarrhoea.*

- *Bouts of vomiting.*

- *Loss or changes in the sense of taste.*

- *Loss or changes in sense of smell (clinical Parosmia or Anosmia (lack of sense of smell).*

- *Sore throat and or difficulties swallowing.*

- *Blood disorders, including new onsets of diabetes and hypertension.*

- *Heartburn (gastroesophageal reflux disease).*

- *Skin rash.*

- *Shortness of breath.*

- *Chest pains.*

- *Palpitations.*

- *Kidney problems (including, acute kidney injury and chronic kidney disease).*

- *Changes in oral health (teeth, saliva, gums).*

- *Tinnitus.*

- *Blood clotting (including deep vein thrombosis and pulmonary embolism).*

- *Erectile dysfunction."*

https://en.wikipedia.org/wiki/Long_COVID

The most common symptoms that persist after 6 months are:

- Fatigue.

- Post-exertional malaise.

- Cognitive dysfunction.

Long COVID and the following conditions are believed to have commonality.

- Chronic fatigue syndrome.

  - https://en.wikipedia.org/wiki/Chronic_fatigue_syndrome

- Cognitive disorder.
  - https://en.wikipedia.org/wiki/Cognitive_disorder
- Multisystem inflammatory syndrome in children.
  - https://en.wikipedia.org/wiki/Multisystem_inflammatory_syndrome_in_children
- Post-Ebola virus syndrome.
  - https://en.wikipedia.org/wiki/Post-Ebola_virus_syndrome
- Post-intensive care syndrome.
  - https://en.wikipedia.org/wiki/Post-intensive_care_syndrome
- Post-polio syndrome.
  - https://en.wikipedia.org/wiki/Post-polio_syndrome
- Post viral cerebellar ataxia.
  - https://en.wikipedia.org/wiki/Post_viral_cerebellar_ataxia

Anyone that is experiencing long COVID should move to a rural green sea level environment as an initial treatment for the condition. An outdoor lifestyle should be adopted. This increases the oxygenation of the human body and will assist in repairing the hypoxic damage that COVID-19 causes.

At the time of publication the following was known about the risk factors for long COVID:

- 1 in 13 adults in the U.S. (7.5%) have long COVID symptoms.
- Nearly three times as many adults ages 50-59 currently have long COVID than those age 80 and older.

- Women are more likely than men to currently have long COVID (9.4% vs. 5.5%).

- Female prevalent symptoms:

  ○ Ear, nose and throat.

  ○ Gastrointestinal.

  ○ Psychiatric and/or mood disorders.

  ○ Neurological.

  ○ Dermatological.

- Male prevalent symptoms:

  ○ Endocrine.

  ○ Renal.

"Long COVID should be suspected in people with unusual failing health."

Steven Magee

Pulse Oximeter

Many people that had the coronavirus experience now own pulse oximeters. Why is this? Because infection with the coronavirus may cause low blood oxygen levels to occur. Remember all of those images of people with coronavirus that we saw on television and in the media? They were being treated with:

- Medical oxygen.

- Continuous positive airway pressure (CPAP) machines.

- Bilevel positive airway pressure (BiPAP) machines.

- Lung ventilators.

- Extracorporeal membrane oxygenation (ECMO) machines. (Last resort!).

These medical treatments all are used to increase the oxygen levels of the blood. Coronavirus damages the lungs to cause these low blood oxygen levels. Some people recover from the lung damage and others do not. "Small Airways Disease" (Bronchiolitis) is becoming a common diagnosis in long COVID survivors. I was medically diagnosed with small airways disease after I started seeking treatment for what I now understand was consistent with long COVID symptoms. Small airways disease has the following characteristics:

- Poor spirometry results.

- Increased lung hyperinflation.

- Poor health.

I had detected low blood oxygen levels with a recording pulse oximeter. They were present during the daytime and the nighttime. It was really bad during sleeping. The medical profession diagnosed the following conditions in me from the medical tests they ran after they saw my pulse oximeter readings:

- Severe Sleep Apnea.

- Positional Sleep Apnea.

- Excessive Daytime Fatigue.

- Air Trapping.

- Asthma.

- Small Airways Disease.

- Depression.

- Delusional Disorder Grandiose.

- Amnesiac Disorder.

- Cognitive Decline.

- Prosopagnosia - Unable to recognize people.

- Fungal Toenails.

- Fecal Urgency.

- Gastrointestinal Polyps.

- Food Intolerance.

As you can see, lung damage can bring on a wide range of health issues. The following recording pulse oximeters were used to monitor my blood oxygen levels:

- Facelake CMS-50E Recording Fingertip Pulse Oximeter. https://www.facelake.com/cms50e.html

- Contec CMS50DA+ Recording Fingertip Pulse Oximeter. https://contechealth.com/collections/pulse-oximeter-1/products/fingertip-pulse-oximeter-usb-cms50da-spo2-monitor-blood-oxygen-24hours-record

You are probably wondering what made me purchase a recording pulse oximeter. I was following up on a chat I had with the nurse that took my blood oxygen readings at the doctors office. I happened to discuss the oxygen reading number and she told me it was lower than most people she saw. The doctor never followed up on this. So I purchased a recording pulse oximeter and discovered I had erratic oxygen levels!

There are two areas that the medical profession considers blood oxygen SpO2 levels to be concerning:

- 92% SpO2 and below: This will get you flagged up for needing further examination and possible medical oxygen treatment.

- 88% SpO2 and below: You will probably be placed onto medical oxygen and admitted to hospital for diagnosis.

On the following pages you will see my pulse oximeter readings from 2015, after my flu-like illness that caused me to start seeking treatment for what I now know to be consistent with long COVID symptoms.

"The medical profession could not diagnose my low blood oxygen levels. It fell onto me to purchase a recording pulse oximeter and detect the erratic blood oxygenation levels."

Steven Magee

2015 SpO2 Sleeping Graph

Severe blood oxygen drops were being seen during sleep. This one dropped to 74% SpO2!

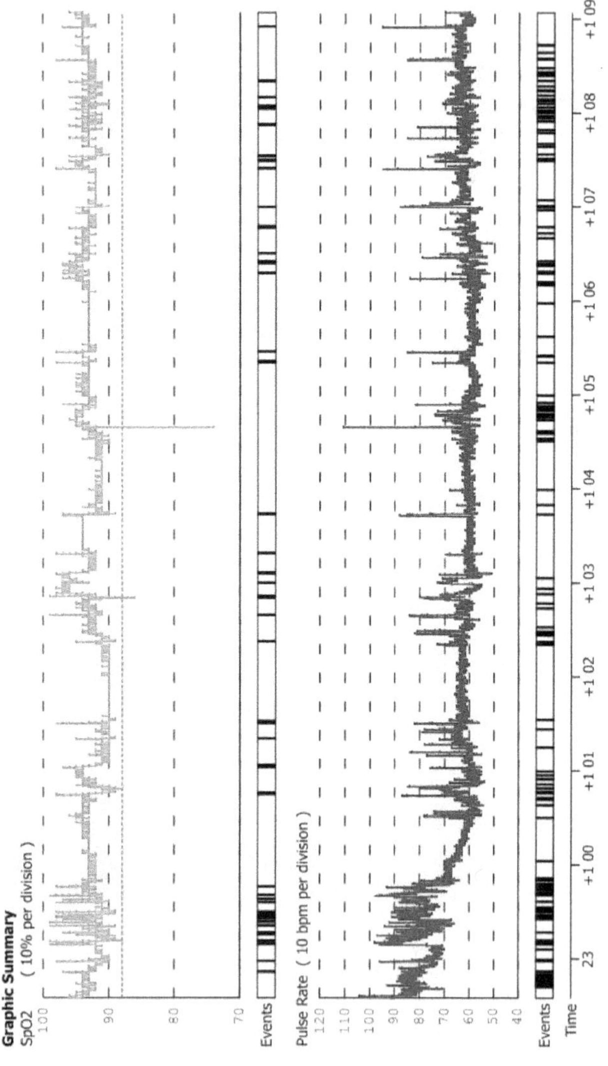

2015 SpO2 Walking Graph

Severe blood oxygen drops were being seen during walking. This one dropped to 75% SpO2!

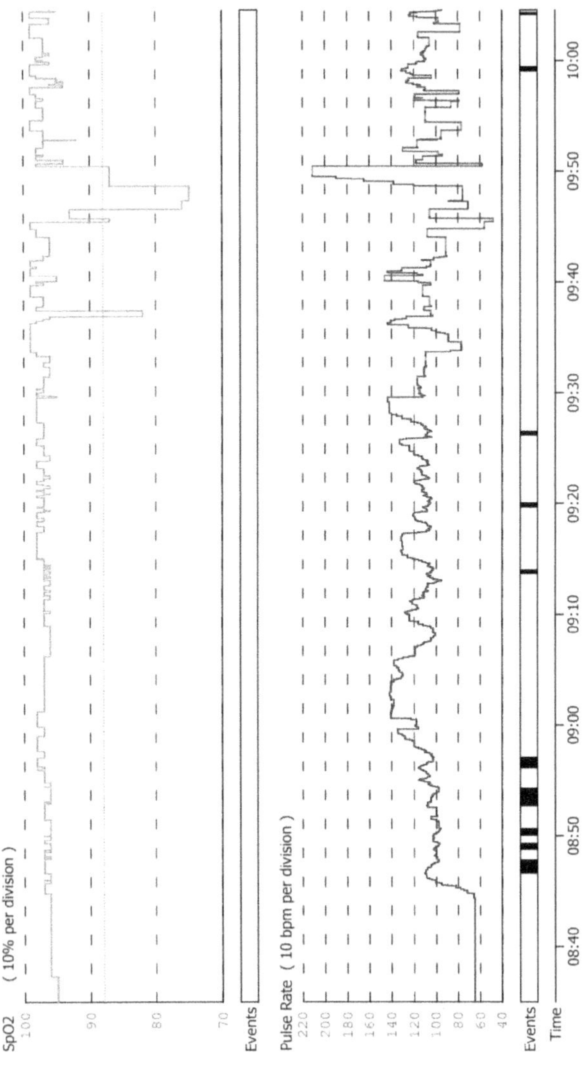

Malnutrition

Coronavirus is known to damage the body, including the organs. Oxygen starvation hypoxic damage may be prevalent throughout the brain and body. Once the brain and body is damaged, you may start to slowly develop malnutrition.

What does malnutrition do to people? The following health conditions are known to occur:

- Food intake:
  - Reduced appetite.
  - Lack of interest in food and drink.
  - Increased appetite as the body looks for missing nutrients.
- Weight:
  - Low weight.
  - Wasting.
  - Loss of fat, muscle mass, and body tissue.
  - Obesity.
- Skin:
  - Pale, thick and dry skin.
  - Bruising easily.
  - Rashes.
  - Changes in skin pigmentation.
- Hair:
  - Thin hair that is tightly curled and pulls out easily.
- Skeletal:
  - Achy joints.

- - Bones that are soft and tender.
- Oral:
  - Gums that bleed easily.
  - Tongue that may be swollen or shriveled and cracked.
- Energy:
  - Feeling tired all the time.
  - Lethargy.
  - Feeling weaker.
- Illness:
  - A higher risk of getting sick and taking longer to heal.
  - Frequent illness.
  - Severe illness as compared to healthy counterparts.
  - Wounds taking a long time to heal.
- Temperature:
  - Feeling cold most of the time.
- Brain:
  - Poor concentration.
  - Low mood.
  - Changes in behavior, such as being unusually irritable, slow or anxious.
- Mental illness:
  - Impaired mental functioning.
  - Anxiety.
  - Depression.
  - Dementia.
  - Schizophrenia.
- Changing senses:

- o   Sight.
- o   Night blindness.
- o   Increased sensitivity to light and glare.
- o   Taste.
- o   Smell.
- o   Dizziness.
- Eating disorders:
  - o   Anorexia nervosa.
  - o   Bulimia nervosa.
- Fertility:
  - o   Infertility issues.
- Children:
  - o   Children not growing or putting on weight at the expected rate.
  - o   Delayed growth in children.
  - o   Short for their age.
- Daily functioning:
  - o   Reduced ability to perform everyday tasks.
- Long term:
  - o   Heart failure.
  - o   Premature death.

Known causes:

- Low food intake.
- Food intolerance.
- Gastrointestinal damage.
- Inflammatory bowel disease.

- Crohn's disease.
- Ulcerative colitis
- Celiac disease.
- Persistent diarrhea.
- Vomiting.
- Organ damage.
- Hypoxia.
- Altitude sickness.
- Radiation exposure.
- Processed foods.
- Restricted diets.
- Alcohol use.
- Drug use.
- Low stomach acid levels.
- Gastrointestinal infections.
- Parasites.
- Poverty.
- Aversion to certain foods.
- Lack of organ meat in the diet.
- Mal-adaptation to the local environment.

There are two types of malnutrition:
- Under-nutrition.
  - Underweight.
  - Skinny.
- Over-nutrition.

- ○ Overweight.
- ○ Obesity.

Both can lead to malnutrition in the body. Malnutrition is a body that is deficient in one or more chemicals or minerals that is needed for normal health. You can be really fat and be in a state of malnutrition!

It was not surprising to see the USA being one of the worst countries in the world for the COVID-19 pandemic. Malnutrition is extensive in the USA, as is mal-adaptation. The USA is predominantly a country of immigrants from all over the world that have no genetic adaptation to the USA! It will be thousands of years before these immigrants develop natural adaptation through many future generations of their family genetics.

It was interesting that during a massive number of doctors visits from 2006 to 2021, I was never referred to a nutritionist! Unfortunately, that is how the USA medical profession works. I am regrettably one the many failures of modern USA medicine.

"Malnutrition is an epidemic in the USA."

Steven Magee

Food Intolerance

Food intolerance is turning into a global pandemic! Lots of people have it and many are misdiagnosed and sickly. The four main types of food intolerance are:

- Gluten.

- Lactose.

- Fructose.

- Protein.

It took many years for me to understand that I had food intolerance and the full extent of it. I initially discovered the gluten, followed by lactose and fructose. It took a few more years to discover the protein intolerance. So I ended up with all four of the main food intolerance types! There was not a lot I could eat by that time. A severely restricted diet from food intolerance may send you into malnutrition! This is how it went for me:

- 2018: Fatigue and sleepiness reaction to eating to pizza. Took gluten out of my diet.

- 2019: Fatigue and sleepiness reaction to milky coffee drinks from the coffee shop. Took lactose out of my diet.

- 2019: Fatigue and sleepiness reaction to fruit smoothie drinks. Took fructose out of my diet.

- 2022: Fatigue and sleepiness reaction to protein drinks, so cut protein out. Treated for protein intolerance with amino acids and all food intolerance disappeared!

Food intolerance typically starts slowly and progresses slowly. It creeps up on you and it is hard to recognize initially. Once you have identified one food intolerance, you may be heading towards the others. Your RADAR needs to be on for all types of food intolerance.

What I did not know was food intolerance can be significantly reduced and even completely eliminated by using nutritional supplements. Today, I eat whatever I like, whenever I like! The nutritional supplementing takes time to work, it typically takes several months to see food intolerance subside. Once subsided, a return to normal eating may take place.

We will look into the nutritional supplements that eliminated food intolerance in me later in the book.

"Food intolerance reactions would make me become very fatigued and sleepy after eating!"

Steven Magee

Urea Cycle Disorders

Coronavirus is known to damage the organs, including the liver and kidneys. Damaged liver and kidneys may produce "Urea Cycle Disorders". A urea cycle disorder can make you really sickly!

It was through researching my protein intolerance that I discovered I probably had an underlying health condition that was causing it. These were the clues:

- Severe reactions to large amounts of protein.

- Suspected hypoxic kidney damage causing protein issues.

- Suspected hypoxic lung damage:
    - Air trapping.
    - Asthma.
    - Small airways disease.

- Beneficial reactions to amino acids.

It did not take long searching the internet to find a rare disease called "Lysinuric Protein Intolerance (LPI)". It causes gastrointestinal issues and malnutrition from loss of amino acids. This comes from the inability to digest the amino acids lysine, arginine, and ornithine. The sickness is known to damage the lungs and kidneys if left untreated. The lung damage the disease causes is called "Pulmonary Alveolar Proteinosis (PAP)". The kidneys develop problems with retaining amino acids, causing amino acid deficiencies within the body. The recommended treatments are:

- Protein be restricted to 0.7–1.2g/kg/day.

- Sodium Benzoate intravenous.

- Calcium supplementation.

- Ornithine supplementation.

- Citrulline be given, limited to 100 mg/kg/day.

- Lysine supplementation (20 mg/kg/day).

- Carnitine supplementation.

- Arginine supplementation.

- Multivitamins.

- Micronutrients.

- Whole-lung lavage to improve respiratory function in persons with pulmonary alveolar proteinosis.

It was interesting that I owned most of the supplements on the above list! Years of experimentation with my health had led me to 80% of the actual treatment! I moved onto the larger treatment with daily doses of L-Citrulline and L-Lysine and saw my health significantly improve!

L-Citrulline and L-Lysine did cause the following symptoms in the first week:

- A dry mouth that slowly subsided.

- Improved digestion. Gas production significantly subsided and I had well formed poops!

- Skull pains were present that subsided. They were comparable to the skull pains that altitude testing had been producing.

- I was seeing foamy urine when urinating.

- A metallic taste in my mouth.

- A sickly feeling, like I was going to vomit in the morning.

- Headaches.

- Constipation.

- Intestinal pains.

- Strong smelling ammonia urine.

- Fatigue.

- Concentration problems with staying on task.

After a couple of weeks the side effects subsided, my body had adapted to the treatment and I was feeling much better.

I did conclude that root cause analysis had correctly identified lysinuric protein intolerance as a significant part of my disease.

Untreated lysinuric protein intolerance can lead to:

- Short stature.

- Muscle weakness.

- Impaired immune function.

- Weak brittle bones (osteoporosis).

- Loose stools or diarrhea.

- Vomiting.

- Feeling sickly and/or fatigued after eating certain foods.

- Anemia.

- Lethargy.

- Lung, kidney, liver, spleen, pancreas and heart problems.

- Pulmonary alveolar proteinosis.

- Breathing problems.

- Low blood oxygen.

- Cognitive impairment.

- Intellectual disability.

- End-stage renal disease.

- Coma.

Regarding amino acids, three are involved in the urea cycle:

- L-Arginine.
- L-Citrulline.
- L-Ornithine.

"I suspected I had a new and undocumented disease and I was not surprised to find a rare disease was part of it!"

Steven Magee

Early Menopause & Manopause

Hypoxic biological damage that coronavirus causes is associated with damage to the human hormone system. That hormone damage may send you into old age far sooner than you expected! Once you have low hormones, you may develop a myriad of adverse conditions.

I remember discussing my health issues with my older female neighbor that had gone through menopause and she stated that everything I was describing about my sickness was consistent with menopause. She was very insightful. She said all of her female friends had similar experiences to mine when they went through menopause!

Early hormone decline in males and females is becoming common and can occur from the following things:

- Chromosomal abnormalities (Fragile X, Turner's syndrome).

- Family history of early or premature menopause (females) or manopause (males).

- Ovaries stop working.

- Testicles stop working.

- Removal of ovaries.

- Removal of testicles.

- Certain infections (tuberculosis, malaria, mumps, coronavirus, COVID-19, Long COVID, and so on).

- Autoimmune diseases:
  - Rheumatoid arthritis.
  - Inflammatory bowel disease.
  - Thyroid disease.

- Chronic fatigue.
- HIV.
- AIDS.
- Radiation exposure.
- Chemical exposure.
- Chemotherapy treatment.
- Radiation treatment.
- Hysterectomy.
- Smoking.
- Shift work.

Long term health issues can be:

- Osteoporosis.
- Cardiovascular disease.
- Physical illness.
- Sexual dysfunction.
- Mental illness.
- Mood disorders.
- Various neurological diseases.
- Increased risk of dementia.
- An earlier death.

Menopause and manopause have different stages:

- Premature menopause and manopause occur before the age of 40. This is called 'Perimenopause' in females.
- Early menopause and manopause occur before age 45.

- Natural menopause and manopause occur around the age of 52.

The defining difference between perimenopause and menopause in females is the absence of periods for at least a year that defines the onset of menopause. Pregnancy can no longer occur in menopause.

Female perimenopause with periods has the following symptoms:

- Sleep disturbances.

- Hot flushes and night sweats.

- Mood changes.

- Anxiety and depression – women will often feel very teary for no apparent reason.

- Weight gain.

- Hair loss.

- Brittle nails.

- Acne.

- Low libido.

- Fatigue.

- Changes in digestion.

- Heavy periods.

Menopause symptoms without periods in females:

- Hot flushes.

- Cold flashes.

- Night sweats.

- Dry skin, eyes and/or mouth.
- Breast tenderness.
- Vaginal dryness.
- Discomfort during sex.
- Changes in libido.
- Urinary urgency.
- Urinary tract infections.
- Racing heart.
- Joint and muscle aches and pains.
- Difficulty sleeping.
- Weight gain.
- Thinning hair.
- Gray hair.
- Hair loss.
- Headaches.
- Low mood.
- Mood swings.
- Anxiety.
- Irritability.
- Depression.
- Concentration problems.
- Memory lapses.
- Reduced sex drive (libido).
- Problems with memory and concentration.

Manopause symptoms in males are similar to above and include:

- Erectile dysfunction.

Treatment in females:

- Combined contraceptive pill.

- Hormone replacement therapy (HRT).

- Certain types of cancer prevent hormone treatment, such as breast cancer.

- Hormone support treatments.

- Amino acids.

- Nutritional supplements to offset aging.

Treatment in males:

- Testosterone.

- Hormone support treatments.

- Amino acids.

- Nutritional supplements to offset aging.

Supplements for treating menopause and manopause will be examined in this book.

"Manopause was causing Altitude Hypersensitivity in me."

Steven Magee

Altitude Hypersensitivity

Coronavirus damages the lungs and many people have been diagnosed with small airways disease after developing long COVID. Damaged lungs can develop pressure sensitivities. This may bring on altitude and weather sensitivities. A low or high pressure weather system passing through your area may make you sick! Changing altitude by flying, driving, vacationing, hiking or skiing may make you sick. Living at altitude may keep you in a permanent state of sickness from altitude sickness health issues. If you are on a CPAP or BiPAP machine, these may may you sickly from the pressurized air they feed to you! If you have had coronavirus, you should be watching for these pressure related health issues!

When I discovered I had altitude hypersensitivity and I was developing altitude sickness at just 1,000 feet, my initial thought was it was probably a life long condition. However, experiments with nutritional supplements in combination with regular altitude exposures were revealing the condition was reducing in severity.

I had a lucky break in this research and that came from my ex-girlfriend. During the relationship, she had been complaining of a lack of sex drive and a lack of interest in sex. She believed she was in menopause. As such, I bought her a menopause support supplement called "Amberen" that was supposed to reduce the symptoms of menopause. However, she refused to take it.

Wondering what to do with the Amberen I now owned, I looked up the formulation and found it had no female hormones in it. It was just a nutritional support supplement. I could see no reason why a man could not take it. A daily dose of Amberen contains a 400mg blend of the following:

- Ammonium Succinate.

- Calcium Disuccinate.

- Monosodium L-Glutamate.

- Glycine.

- Magnesium Disuccinate.

- Zinc Difumarate.

- Tocopheryl Acetate.

The manufacturer states: *"Amberen contains a proprietary blend of bioactive antioxidants, amino acids, minerals and vitamin E."*

So I started to take it in June 2022. A week after taking the Amberen, I did an altitude test. I took my body up from 600 feet above sea level to 4,024 feet and much to my surprise noticed no symptoms that could make a diagnosis of altitude hypersensitivity. A few days later I took my body from 140 feet above sea level to 6,632 feet and again saw no symptoms that could make a diagnosis of altitude hypersensitivity.

This was the first time this had occurred during altitude testing. The Amberen had changed the body chemistry. I had noticed nerve pains in my face accompanied by twitching since I had been taking this supplement, so something was changing in the body regarding the nervous system.

The Amberen had fixed things! Why was this? Because I was age 52, I was in "Manopause". Manopause is the male equivalent of the female menopause. Just like aged females, the hormones also change in men after forty years of age. Hormone decline occurs in both sexes after age forty. But was there any evidence it could be the Amberen?

I took a look at the Amberen website and found this statement: *"Glycine: An amino acid involved in the processes regulating brain-cell activity. In combination with magnesium, it makes brain mitochondria more resistant to low-oxygen conditions (hypoxia), which, in turn, results in the normalization of the psycho-emotional balance in the body."*

https://amberen.com/am-ingredients

So one of the ingredients of Amberen is a known treatment for hypoxia! I was right! Increasing altitude causes hypoxia and glycine treats it. To confirm the information was correct on the Amberen website, I did an internet search on "glycine altitude" and found numerous articles about its beneficial effects at altitude.

After one month of taking Amberen:

- Regular altitude testing from sea level up to 6,632 feet was showing no evidence of altitude hypersensitivity.

- The side effects were:
  - Nerve pains in my face.
  - Facial muscles twitching.
  - Insomnia.
  - Mild headaches.
  - Mild heart pains.
  - All side effects subsided after one month of Amberen administration.

Amberen treats altitude hypersensitivity. Altitude hypersensitivity at 1,000 feet returned during minimum supplement testing and this indicated it was one of the removed supplements that was causing it. Reviewing my notes indicated that it had followed the removal of Acetyl-L-Carnitine HCI. Taking L-Carnitine L-Tartrate at 500mg daily cleared up the altitude hypersensitivity.

Why did I switch from Acetyl-L-Carnitine HCI to L-Carnitine L-Tartrate? I could not purchase Acetyl-L-Carnitine HCI at the time, due to the COVID-19 pandemic shortages. L-Carnitine L-Tartrate was the closest thing to it that was available for purchase.

The question arose of what was the minimum amount of supplements needed to prevent altitude hypersensitivity from occurring? I removed all supplements with the exception of

Amberen and L-Carnitine L-Tartrate and continued to be free of altitude hypersensitivity. I did see some adverse reactions to L-Carnitine L-Tartrate as I raised the dose to 500 mg 4 times daily (total 2,000 mg daily):

- Day 1: No symptoms.

- Day 2: Hungry all day long and overeating.

- Day 3: Fatigued all day long and stayed in bed. Low appetite.

- Day 4: Mating cycle was triggered during morning sleep. Woke up at sunrise. Headache all day long. Stayed in bed most of the day.

- Day 5: Milder headache and lethargic. In bed in the afternoon with headache. The headache seemed to increase as I was taking the four doses of L-Carnitine L-Tartrate during the day. Right earache during the evening that subsided by bedtime.

- Day 6: Mild headache that subsided by lunchtime. Afternoon fatigue. Altitude test to 4,024 feet. No symptoms of altitude hypersensitivity. Sore right knee joint when walking in the evening.

- Day 7: Woke up energized. Fatigue onset as the day progressed that did not respond to caffeine. Hungry in the evening and overeating.

- Day 8: Woke up at sunrise. Fatigued and exhibiting confusion. Altitude test to 6,632 feet. No symptoms of altitude hypersensitivity. Ears popping and skull pains.

- Day 9: Feeling fine.

The dose was raised to what the manufacturer recommended, as I was concerned that I may not be taking enough of it to fully treat the altitude hypersensitivity. Based on the above symptoms, there was a profound response to the increased dosing which I took as an indication that a deficiency was being corrected in the body.

I removed the Amberen to see if the L-Carnitine L-Tartrate could treat altitude hypersensitivity on its own.

Research into L-Carnitine L-Tartrate indicated that 3,000 mg is considered the safe level of maximum dosing in adults. Given the profound reactions I was having to it, I decided to do a couple of weeks at 3 doses daily of 1,000 mg. The following reactions were seen at the maximum dosing level:

- Day 1: Insomnia until 1 am.

- Day 2: Woke up fatigued. Coffee cleared it. Had good energy levels and concentration.

- Day 3: Had good energy levels and concentration.

- Day 4: Fatigued PM.

- Day 5: Feeling fine. Altitude test to 2,000 feet. No symptoms of altitude hypersensitivity.

- Day 6: Feeling fine.

- Day 7 to 10: Started to develop mild headaches.

- Day 11: Altitude test to 4,024 feet. Mild headache that progressed into severe headache at altitude. Showing increasing confusion during the drive. Started Amberen to treat the headache and confusion. Both subsided during sleep.

- Day 12: At 140 feet above sea level. Fatigued in the morning that responded to caffeine.

- Day 13: Altitude test to 6,632 feet. Feeling normal. Mild headache during altitude exposure. Cleared up at sea level in Kona. No further issues on the drive home at 1,000 to 2,000 feet. Slept at 600 feet.

- Day 14: Mild skull pains.

- Day 15: Back to normal.

Removing Amberen did cause altitude hypersensitivity to return. It was also accompanied by headaches. Taking the Amberen cleared up both conditions. It appears the altitude exposure is needed for nutritional absorption throughout the body, including the brain.

There appears to be two supplements needed to keep altitude hypersensitivity treated once it has been cleared and that is:

- L-Carnitine L-Tartrate at 500 mg to 3,000 mg daily.

  - Bulk Supplements.

- Amberen.

  - Biogix, Inc.

L-Carnitine and Amberen were working together to clear up the altitude hypersensitivity. There is an interaction taking place between them and one does not work without the other.

I have remained free of most food intolerance using only L-Carnitine L-Tartrate. Mental and physical health were good. Energy levels were good.

Regarding the rest of the supplements, it seems they reduce the altitude hypersensitivity, but they do not fully clear it up like the L-Carnitine and Amberen do. Given the rest of the supplements improve sex, it appears they are treating deficiencies within the body.

The key suspected ingredients that treat altitude hypersensitivity were L-Carnitine and glycine. Research revealed a supplement that had both of these in it called "Glycine Propionyl-L-Carnitine (GPLC)". I purchased the following GPLC products:

- Carlyle GPLC Supplement 1250mg.

  - Propionyl-L-Carnitine 824 mg.

  - Glycine 282 mg.

  - CoQ10 60 mg.

- VitaMonk GlycoTrax.
    - Glycine Propionyl-L-Carnitine 1,000 mg.

L-Carnitine and Amberen were removed and were replaced by GPLC. My body remained free of altitude hypersensitivity during altitude tests. I took GPLC for three months and did not see altitude hypersensitivity return during that time.

There was a notable difference in the GPLC supplements. Carlyle GPLC was unstable and would degrade after opening the supplement container. When I would put it in my pill box, by the end of a week the Carlyle GPLC capsules would be degrading. After a couple of months in the pill bottle, they were unusable. I threw the last few capsules I had away. No such issues were observed with VitaMonk GlycoTrax. The Carlyle GPLC appeared to be the better GPLC supplement for treating altitude hypersensitivity and this reflected its higher level of GPLC.

These are my conclusions about treating my altitude hypersensitivity:

1. Low protein organic diet.

2. Base nutritional supplements are L-Carnitine and glycine.

3. Optimized nutrition through appropriate supplementation and diet.

There is currently no known cure for altitude hypersensitivity, it appears to be a lifelong treatment. It may be arising in the general population from flying, mountain activities, living at altitude, lung damage, man-made environmental changes, climate change and new bacteria and viruses.

"I was surprised at how simple the treatment for Altitude Hypersensitivity was."

Steven Magee

Fungal Infections

Coronavirus is known to damage the human immune system. Once you have a damaged immune system, you will become vulnerable to a wide variety of infections. One of these is systemic fungal infections. I noticed after my flu-like sickness that my big toenails that always had issues since my late thirties were now growing thick and discolored. The medical profession tested the nails and informed me that I had a "Onychomycosis" fungal infection.

The Wikipedia article *"Onychomycosis"* states: *"Onychomycosis, also known as tinea unguium, is a fungal infection of the nail. Symptoms may include white or yellow nail discoloration, thickening of the nail, and separation of the nail from the nail bed. Toenails or fingernails may be affected, but it is more common for toenails. Complications may include cellulitis of the lower leg. A number of different types of fungus can cause onychomycosis, including dermatophytes and Fusarium. Risk factors include athlete's foot, other nail diseases, exposure to someone with the condition, peripheral vascular disease, and poor immune function. The diagnosis is generally suspected based on the appearance and confirmed by laboratory testing. Onychomycosis does not necessarily require treatment. The antifungal medication terbinafine taken by mouth appears to be the most effective but is associated with liver problems. Trimming the affected nails when on treatment also appears useful. There is a ciclopirox-containing nail polish, but there is no evidence that it works. The condition returns in up to half of cases following treatment. Not using old shoes after treatment may decrease the risk of recurrence. Onychomycosis occurs in about 10 percent of the adult population, with older people more frequently affected. Males are affected more often than females. Onychomycosis represents about half of nail disease. It was first determined to be the result of a fungal infection in 1853 by Georg Meissner."*

https://en.wikipedia.org/wiki/Onychomycosis

For me, it was a slowly progressing condition that started in my late thirties. Initially my big toenails would spontaneously fall off for no reason and then regrow back. It progressed into them discoloring. Then they became thick and ugly after my long COVID symptoms developed! That is when I was referred to the clinic that diagnosed onychomycosis. My toenails were surgically removed, but they grew back the same! I gave up on fixing them!

Then I started recovering my health and started to realize that during the time I had the strange toenail issues, I had systemic ammonia poisoning from the urea cycle disorder. It was unlikely that the toenails would ever clear up while that was present. So once the systemic poisoning was treated, it was time to revisit my fungal toenails again!

The first attempt to clear them up was by painting tea tree oil onto them every day. That never worked. Then I came across stories of people painting vitamin E onto their nails and clearing it up. I also came across information that stated the most successful treatment was to take oral anti-fungal medication for several months.

As such, I decided to take a high dose of Vitamin E at the same time as painting the nails with Vitamin E. I was using the high dose of oral vitamin E as an oral anti-fungal. I threw in 10,000 mcg of biotin also, as it was known to fix nail issues. Vitamin C was a known anti-fungal, so I took 2,000 mg. This is what I was doing daily:

- Paint all toenails with vitamin E after showering.

- Take 8 capsules of 180 mg vitamin E (Total 1,440 mg).

- 10,000 mcg Biotin.

- 2,000 mg vitamin C.

I was creating an internal systemic environment of anti-fungals as well as painting an anti-fungal directly onto all toenails. What happened? I saw improved hair and nail growth!

Risk factors for fungal nails are:

- Advancing age (usually over the age of 60).

- Diminished blood circulation.

- Longer exposure to fungi.

- Nails which grow more slowly and thicken.

- Reduced immune function increasing susceptibility to infection.

- Nail fungus tends to affect men more often than women and is associated with a family history of this infection.

- Perspiring heavily.

- A humid or moist environment.

- Psoriasis.

- Wearing socks and shoes that hinder ventilation and do not absorb perspiration.

- Going barefoot in damp public places such as swimming pools, gyms and shower rooms.

- Having athlete's foot (tinea pedis).

- Skin or nail injury.

- Damaged nail.

- Infection.

- Diabetes.

- Circulation problems.

- Weakened immune system.

Other treatments that are known to work are:

- Snakeroot (Ageratina pichinchensis) extract applied to the nails daily.

- Vicks VapoRub applied to the nails daily.

What I did not know when I had this experience was fungal nails were symptomatic of a declining immune system. Until my immune system was fixed, it was unlikely that my fungal nail infection would be treatable! The doctors never made this connection when I was under their care.

"Nutritional supplements improved my fungal toenails more than the doctors could!"

Steven Magee

My Health Conditions

I successfully treated a variety of health conditions during developing pandemic supplements:

- Severe Sleep Apnea.
  - Treated by moving to a rural environment near to sea level in 2021. Take magnesium. No sleeping on the back. No need for a sleep apnea machine.

- Lysinuric Protein Intolerance.
  - Treated in spring 2022.

- Food Intolerance.
  - Treated in summer 2022.

- Altitude Hypersensitivity.
  - Treated in fall 2022.

- Onychomycosis.
  - Currently being treated by oral and topical vitamin E in spring 2023. Early signs of improved nail and hair growth are being seen.

Nutritional supplements had a profound effect on the above conditions. As you can see from the above, once you find the correct supplements for one condition successfully, that often snowballs into finding the supplements for your other health issues also.

Most mental and physical health conditions cleared up as pandemic supplements was being developed during 2021 to 2023.

"Aging may take you journeying through a variety of health conditions."

Steven Magee

49

<u>Overview Of Pandemic Supplements</u>

The following chapters will look into the various supplements that were used in the formulations of pandemic supplements. It was a process that was driven by health conditions being uncovered, side effects, toxicity and modern society to produce three distinctly different formulations. They all stopped altitude hypersensitivity, food intolerance and lysinuric protein intolerance from occurring.

You will notice that I had high dosed with some supplements, sometimes higher than the upper limit that is known to cause side effects. That is because I know I have nutrient absorption issues and often cannot fully absorb the nutritional supplement. In cases where the body is deficient in a nutritional supplement, it can take several months of high dosing to eliminate a nutritional deficiency.

When high dosing, I monitor my health for adverse side effects and reduce the dosing of the suspected supplement whenever I see it.

This listing is not a comprehensive look into supplements, but rather a list I was using to monitor specific supplements that I was interested in and was using. Comprehensive listings of supplements are available on the internet and in books.

Interactions with prescription medications and medical treatments were not looked into, as I do not use any.

You will see "RDA" frequently, it is the recommended dietary allowance. It is a guide to how much to take on a daily basis for most healthy people.

"Developing supplement protocols requires watching for health improvements, side effects, toxicity and societal prejudices."

Steven Magee

Multivitamin

The multivitamin is the base for supplementation. Depending on your particular health conditions, you may need to be taking other supplements in addition to it.

When buying a multivitamin, it is important to read the supplement label to find out what it contains. There are so many different types of multivitamins available because they have so many different formulations!

I chose "Kirkland Signature Daily Multi" for my base multivitamin due to its large range of included nutritional supplements. It has an excellent review rating of 4.6 out of 5. It contains:

- Vitamin A 1,050 mcg (117% RDA).

- Vitamin C 90 mg (100% RDA).

- Vitamin D 10 mcg / 400 IU (50% RDA).

- Vitamin E 13.5 mg (90% RDA).

- Vitamin K 25 mcg (21% RDA).

- Vitamin B1 Thiamin 1.5 mg (125% RDA).

- Vitamin B2 Riboflavin 1.7 mg (131% RDA).

- Niacin 20 mg (125% RDA).

- Vitamin B6 2 mg (118%RDA).

- Folate 833 mcg DFE (500 mcg folic acid) (208% RDA).

- Vitamin B12 6 mcg (250% RDA).

- Biotin 30 mcg (100% RDA).

- Panthothenic acid 10 mg (200% RDA).

- Calcium 200 mg (15% RDA).

- Iron 18 mg (100%).

- Phosphorus 109 mg (9% RDA).

- Iodine 150 mcg (100% RDA).

- Magnesium 100 mg (24% RDA).

- Zinc 11 mg (100% RDA).

- Selenium 55 mcg (100% RDA).

- Copper 0.9 mg (100% RDA).

- Manganese 2.3 mg (100% RDA).

- Chromium 35 mcg (100% RDA).

- Molybdenum 45 mcg (100% RDA).

- Chloride 72 mg (3% RDA).

- Potassium 80 mg (2% RDA).

- Silicon 2 mg.

- Lycopine 300 mcg.

- Lutein 250 mcg.

- Boron 150 mcg.

- Vanadium 10 mcg.

- Nickel 5 mcg.

"When you are sick, a good multivitamin is always a great starting point."

Steven Magee

B Vitamins

B vitamins are often called "Energy Vitamins". You will commonly see B vitamins in energy drinks. Like the multivitamin, there are many different formulations of B vitamin supplements. The formulation that was used in the book was "CVS Health Super B Complex With Vitamin C" which has a 4.5 out of 5 review rating. It contains:

- Vitamin C Ascorbic Acid 60 mg (100% RDA).

- Vitamin B1 Thiamin Mononitrate 25 mg (1,667% RDA).

- Vitamin B2 Riboflavin 20mg (1,176% RDA).

- Naicin as Niacinamide 25mg (125% RDA).

- Vitamin B6 Pyrodoxine Hydrochloride 5 mg (250% RDA).

- Folic Acid 400 mcg (100% RDA).

- Vitamin B12 Cyanocobalamin 100 mcg (1,667 RDA).

- Biotin as d-Biotin 1,000 mcg (333% RDA).

- Pantothenic Acid as d-Calcium Pantothenate 5.5 mg (55% RDA).

"B vitamins are a key component of my nutritional supplementation protocol."

Steven Magee

Vitamin B6

Vitamin B6 is an important B vitamin that has many functions in the body.

Functions:

- Brain development.

- Nervous system.

- Immune system.

- Prevents anemia.

- Enzyme functionality.

- Protein metabolism.

- Maintaining normal levels of homocysteine.

- Gluconeogenesis.

- Glycogenolysis.

- Hemoglobin formation.

- May prevents kidney stones.

- May reduce female premenstrual syndrome (PMS) symptoms.

Deficiency symptoms:

- Confusion.

- Depression.

- Weakened immune system.

- Microcytic anemia.

- Electroencephalographic abnormalities.

- Dermatitis with cheilosis.

- Glossitis.

- Infants: Irritability, abnormally acute hearing, and convulsive seizures.

Reported side effects:

- Nausea.

- Stomach pain.

- Loss of appetite.

- Headaches.

Toxicity:

- Skin lesions.

- Heartburn.

- Photosensitivity.

- Reduced ability to sense pain or extreme temperatures.

- Ataxia.

- Nausea.

- Brain problems.

- Nerve problems.

- Neuropathy.

RDA:

- Adults: 1.3 mg.

- Elderly 50+: Males: 1.7 mg. Females: 1.5 mg.

Tolerable upper intake level:

- Adults: 100 mg.

"*Too much vitamin B6 may cause nerve issues.*"

Steven Magee

<u>Biotin (B7)</u>

Biotin is commonly taken to form strong hair and nails.

Functions:

- Helps enzymes to break down fats, carbohydrates, and proteins.

- Forms glucose.

- Regulates signals sent by cells.

- Gene activity.

- Reduces hypoglycemia.

- Reduces hyperlipidemia.

- Glucose control.

- May reduce diabetic nerve pain.

- May reduce multiple sclerosis.

Deficiency symptoms:

- Thinning hair.

- Hair loss.

- Scaly skin rashes around eyes, nose, mouth and perineum.

- Conjunctivitis.

- Ketolactic acidosis.

- Aciduria.

- Skin problems.

- Biotin deficiency facies.

- Brittle nails.
- Nail problems.
- High cholesterol.
- Heart problems.
- Seizures.
- Skin infection.
- Depression.
- Lethargy.
- Exhaustion.
- Hallucinations.
- Paresthesias of the extremities.
- Numbness and tingling in arms and legs.
- Hypotonia, lethargy, and developmental delay in infants.
- Biotinidase deficiency.

Reported side effects:
- Stomach ache.
- Digestive upset.
- Insomnia.
- Excessive thirst.
- Insulin problems.
- Kidney problems.

RDA:
- Adults: 30 mcg.
- Lactation: 35 mcg.

Tolerable upper intake level:

- No upper limit is known.

"People take biotin in huge doses to improve their hair and nails."

Steven Magee

<u>Folate (B9)</u>

Folate has a variety of names and is also known as folacin, folic acid and vitamin B9. It is often taken by pregnant women and people who eat grain products, as it is added to grains during manufacturing.

Functions:

- Forms DNA.

- Forms RNA.

- Protein metabolism.

- Breaks down homocysteine.

- Red blood cell production.

- Fetal development during pregnancy.

- May reduce autism spectrum disorder (ASD).

- May prevent cancer before it has formed.

Deficiency symptoms:

- Elevated blood concentrations of homocysteine.

- Megaloblastic anemia.

- Irritability.

- Headache.

- Shortness of breath.

- Weakness.

- Fatigue.

- Heart palpitations.

- Irregular heartbeat.

- Shortness of breath.

- Difficulty concentrating.

- Hair loss.

- Changes in skin, hair, or fingernail pigmentation.

- Gastrointestinal symptoms.

- Pale skin.

- Mouth sores.

- Soreness in the tongue.

- Birth defects of the spine (spina bifida).

- Birth defects of the brain (anencephaly).

- Increased risk of heart disease.

- Increased risk of stroke.

- Depression.

- Poor response to antidepressants.

- May increase the risk of dementia.

- May increase the risk of Alzheimer's disease.

- Low infant birth weight.

- Preterm delivery.

- Fetal growth retardation.

- Neural tube defects (NTD).

Reported side effects:

- May speed up gastrointestinal polyp growth.

- May increase the risk of colon cancer.

- May hide the symptoms of B12 deficiency.

- May damage the brain and nervous system in people with untreated B12 deficiency.

- May promote cancer that is pre-existing.

RDA:

- Adults: 400 mcg.

- Pregnancy: 600 mcg.

- Lactating: 500 mcg.

- Adults regularly drinking alcohol: 600 mcg.

Tolerable upper intake level:

- 1,000 mcg.

"Birth defects dropped in the general population after folate was added to grain products."

Steven Magee

Vitamin B12

Vitamin B12 is associated with boosting energy levels. To do so, it is generally taken in huge doses. I was testing low on vitamin B12. When it was low, I was experiencing a strange feeling of someone being in the room with me, even though I was alone. It cleared up after high dosing with vitamin B12 and D.

There is little information on the toxicity of vitamin B12. It is widely regarded as being tolerated by the human body in large doses. I have taken it at 20,000 mcg daily in the past when trying to raise up my low vitamin B12 levels. I definitely felt better once I moved my vitamin B12 from the low to the high range of the medical testing.

When I told one of my doctors about my improved health on vitamin B12, he told me everyone perks up when they take vitamin B12! Curiously, he had never prescribed it to me or told me to take it!

Function:

- Required for the development, myelination, and function of the central nervous system.

- Healthy red blood cell formation.

- DNA synthesis.

- Functions as a cofactor for two enzymes, methionine synthase and L-methylmalonyl-CoA mutase.

- Improves anemia.

- Increased energy levels.

- Better mental functioning.

Deficiency symptoms:

- Pernicious anemia.

- Megaloblastic anemia (characterized by large, abnormally nucleated red blood cells).

- Low counts of white and red blood cells, platelets, or a combination.

- Glossitis of the tongue.

- Fatigue.

- Intestinal problems.

- Palpitations.

- Pale skin.

- Mood disturbances.

- Depression.

- Dementia.

- Weight loss.

- Infertility.

- Neurological changes, such as numbness and tingling in the hands and feet.

- Nerve damage.

- Muscle weakness.

- In pregnant and breastfeeding women, vitamin B12 deficiency might cause neural tube defects, developmental delays, failure to thrive, and anemia in offspring.

Reported side effects:

- Headache.

- Nausea and vomiting.

- Diarrhea.

- Fatigue or weakness.

- Tingling sensation in hands and feet.

RDA:

- Adults: 2.4 mcg.

Tolerable upper intake level:

- No upper limit has been established.

"Pernicious anemia killed many people before the development of B12 supplements!"

Steven Magee

Vitamin C

Vitamin C is commonly associated with preventing or reducing the severity of colds and flu. It is called ascorbic acid and is commonly found in citrus fruits. Historically, it was used to prevent scurvy from developing in sailors.

Functions:

- Forms blood vessels, cartilage, muscle and collagen in bones.

- Antioxidant.

- Assists iron absorption.

- Prevents age-related macular degeneration (AMD) from worsening.

- Lower risk of developing cataracts.

- Topical application:
  - Stimulates collagen production.
  - Protects against damage from ultraviolet (UV) sunlight.

Deficiency symptoms:

- Scurvy:
  - Skin spots caused by bleeding and bruising from broken blood vessels.
  - Swelling or bleeding of gums, and eventual loss of teeth.
  - Hair loss.
  - Delayed healing of skin wounds.

- Fatigue.
- Malaise.
- Iron-deficiency anemia.

Reported side effects:

- Nausea.
- Vomiting.
- Diarrhea.
- Heartburn.
- Stomach cramps.
- Bloating.
- Fatigue.
- Sleepiness.
- Insomnia.
- Headache.
- Skin flushing.

Toxicity:

- Gastrointestinal distress, diarrhea and kidney stones may occur at excessive levels.

RDA:

- Adults 19 years and older: Male: 90 mg. Female 75 mg.
- Pregnancy: 85 mg.
- Lactation: 120 mg.
- Smokers: Additional 35 mg.

Tolerable upper intake level:

- 2,000mg daily.

"Vitamin C prevented scurvy in sailors."

Steven Magee

Vitamin D

Vitamin D is often called the "Sunlight Vitamin", as it is produced when the body is exposed to sunlight. I have tried to raise my extremely low vitamin D levels by sunbathing, but it had minimal effect. I eventually had to do high dose supplementation for several months to get my vitamin D to go from the low level to the high level of the medical testing range.

When it was low, I was experiencing a strange feeling of someone being in the room with me, even though I was alone. It cleared up after high dosing with vitamin B12 and D.

Functions:

- Calcium absorption.

- Bone strength.

- Strong teeth.

- Anti-inflammatory.

- Antioxidant.

- Neuro-protective.

- Immunity.

- Muscle function.

- Brain cell activity.

- Reduces the risk of multiple sclerosis.

- Prevents rickets.

Deficiency symptoms:

- Cognitive decline.

- Bone disorders.

- Multiple sclerosis.

- Osteomalacia.

- Osteoporosis.

- Psoriasis.

- Rickets.

Reported side effects:

- Nausea.

- Vomiting.

- Poor appetite.

- Weight loss.

- Constipation.

- Weakness.

- Confusion.

- Disorientation.

- Heart rhythm problems.

- Kidney stones.

- Kidney damage.

RDA:

- 400 IU for children up to age 12 months.

- 600 IU for people ages 1 to 70 years.

- 800 IU for people over 70 years.

Tolerable upper intake level:

- 4,000 IU.

72

"High doses of vitamin D for several months were needed to move from the low end of the medical testing range to the high end."

Steven Magee

Vitamin E

Vitamin E is known for its anti-fungal properties. People have been regularly painting it onto their fungal nail infections and clearing them up. It also has protective properties from ultra-violet (UV) light. I have taken 1,440 mg daily for several months without any apparent negative issues after the initial adjustment to it.

Function:

- Antioxidant.

- Anti-fungal.

- Potentially anti-aging.

- Blood thinner.

- Widens blood vessels.

- Reduces the risk of blood clots.

- Strengthens hair, skin, and nails.

- Protective against ultraviolet (UV) light.

- May delay the progression of Alzheimer's disease.

- May improve fatty liver disease.

- May improve atopic dermatitis.

Deficiency symptoms:

- Nerve pain (neuropathy).

Reported side effects:

- Increased risk of bleeding.

- Potentially fatal bleeding.

- Interferes with blood clotting.

- Increased risk of hemorrhagic stroke.

- Nausea.

- Diarrhea.

- Intestinal cramps.

- Fatigue.

- Weakness.

- Headache.

- Blurred vision.

- Rash.

- Gonadal dysfunction.

- Increased concentration of creatine in the urine (creatinuria).

- May increase the risk of prostate cancer.

- High doses may increase the risk of death.

RDA:

- Adults: 15 mg.

- Breastfeeding: 19 mg.

Tolerable upper intake level:

- Adults: 1,000 mg.

"High doses of vitamin E gave me looser stools!"

Steven Magee

Metals

The human body requires numerous metals in the diet to be healthy. Some of these are iron, magnesium, and zinc. There are many metals the body needs to be in good health. Deficiencies will bring on poor health and too much may bring on toxicity symptoms. Numerous metals are considered essential to the human diet:

1. Sodium (Na).

2. Potassium (K).

3. Magnesium (Mg).

4. Calcium (Ca).

5. Manganese (Mn).

6. Iron (Fe).

7. Cobalt (Co).

8. Copper (Cu).

9. Zinc (Zn).

10. Molybdenum (Mo).

11. Vanadium (V).

12. Chromium (Cr)

13. Manganese (Mn).

14. Nickel (Ni).

15. Cadmium (Cd).

Deficiencies of metals are known to cause:

- Neurological disorders (Alzheimer's, Parkinson's and Huntington's disorders).

- Mental health issues.

- Cardiovascular diseases.

- Cancer

- Diabetes.

- Anemia.

Iron deficient anemia is the most common metal disease in the global population. Metal deficiency is linked to the following diseases:

- Iron and cobalt - anemia.

- Copper - brain, heart diseases and anemia.

- Zinc - growth retardation and skin changes.

- Calcium - bone deterioration.

- Chromium - reduces glucose tolerance.

We will look into the ones I identified as needing supplementation in my diet in the coming chapters.

"Too little or too much metal in the diet can make you sick!"

Steven Magee

<u>Calcium</u>

Calcium is commonly associated with bone growth and teeth. Milk products are the typical dietary source.

Function:

- Bone health.

- Teeth health.

- Blood clotting.

- Muscles contraction.

- Heart rhythms.

- Nerve function.

- Hormone function.

- Lowers blood pressure.

- May protect against colorectal cancer.

Deficiency symptoms:

- Muscle cramps or weakness.

- Numbness or tingling in fingers.

- Abnormal heart rate.

- Poor appetite.

- Osteopenia.

- Osteoporosis.

Reported side effects:

- Increased cardiovascular disease.

- Rickets in children.

Toxicity:

- Hypercalcemia.

- Blood may clot.

- Arteries may harden.

RDA:

- Adults: Male 1,000 mg. Female: 1,000 mg.

- Elderly: Male 71+ 1,200 mg. Female 51+ 1,200 mg.

- Pregnancy and lactating: 1,000 mg.

Tolerable upper intake level:

- 2,500 mg.

"I get my calcium from milk, yogurt and cheese."

Steven Magee

<u>Iron</u>

Iron deficiency is a global pandemic. It is the most common of the metal deficiencies. Females are affected the most due to blood loss that periods cause every month. It is important when comparing males to females that you are aware that the female engages in monthly bloodletting through periods that does not occur in males. It is widely acknowledged that females live longer than males and this monthly iron loss through bleeding is thought to be a factor in their longevity.

Function:

- Creates healthy blood cells.

- Prevents anemia.

- Brain development.

- Growth.

- Cell production.

- Hormone production.

Deficiency symptoms:

- Extreme fatigue.

- Lightheadeness.

- Weakness.

- Confusion.

- Loss of concentration.

- Sensitivity to cold.

- Shortness of breath.

- Rapid heartbeat.

- Pale skin.

- Hair loss.

- Brittle nails.

- Pica: cravings for dirt, clay, ice, or other non-food items.

Reported side effects:

- Backache, groin, side, or muscle pain.

- Chest pain.

- Chills.

- Dizziness.

- Fainting.

- Fast heartbeat.

- Fever with increased sweating.

- Flushing.

- Headache.

- Metallic taste.

- Nausea or vomiting.

- Numbness, pain, or tingling of hands or feet.

- Pain or redness at injection site.

- Redness of skin.

- Skin rash or hives.

- Swelling of mouth or throat.

- Troubled breathing.

- Abdominal or stomach pain.

- Cramping or soreness.
- Double vision.
- General unwell feeling.
- Weakness without feeling dizzy or faint.
- Chest or throat pain, especially when swallowing.
- Stools with signs of blood (red or black color).
- Constipation
- Diarrhea.
- Leg cramps.
- Nausea.
- Vomiting.
- Darkened urine.
- Heartburn.
- Stained teeth.

Toxicity:

- Constipation.
- Diarrhea (may contain blood).
- Fever.
- Nausea.
- Stomach pain or cramping (sharp).
- Abdominal pain.
- Vomiting, severe (may contain blood).
- Bluish-colored lips, fingernails, and palms of hands.
- Convulsions (seizures).

- Pale, clammy skin.

- Shallow and rapid breathing.

- Unusual tiredness or weakness.

- Weak and fast heartbeat.

RDA:

- Adolescents 14-18 years: Males: 11 mg. Females: 15 mg.

- Adults: Males 8 mg. Females 18 mg.

- Elderly females after menopause: 8 mg.

- Pregnancy: 27 mg.

- Lactation: 9 mg.

Tolerable upper intake level:

- Children: 40 mg.

- 14+ years of age: 45 mg.

"Iron deficiency is the most common of the nutritional metal deficiencies in humans."

Steven Magee

<u>Magnesium</u>

Magnesium is known for its positive effects on sleep disorders. It can stop grinding of the teeth and improve the sleep cycle. In me, it did both.

Functions:

- Antacid.

- Laxative.

- Building proteins.

- Enzyme functioning.

- Strong bones.

- Regulating blood sugar.

- Blood pressure.

- Muscle function.

- Nerve function.

- Steady heart beat.

- Raises vitamin D levels.

- Prevents leg and foot cramps.

- Prevents clogged arteries.

- Prevents strokes.

- Prevents heart disease.

- Prevents diabetes.

- Reduces stress.

- Reduces anxiety.

- Improves mood.

- Improves sleep.

- Reduces teeth grinding at night.

Deficiency symptoms:

- Fatigue.

- Weakness.

- Poor appetite.

- Nausea.

- Vomiting

- Numbness or tingling in skin.

- Muscle cramps.

- Seizures.

- Abnormal heart rate.

- Migraine headaches.

- Depression.

- Alzheimer's disease.

- High blood pressure.

- Strokes.

- Diabetes.

- Heart disease.

- Osteoporosis.

Reported side effects:

- Stomach upset.

- Nausea.

- Vomiting.
- Abdominal cramping.
- Diarrhea.

Toxicity:

- Diarrhea.
- Nausea.
- Vomiting
- Cramping.
- Low mood.
- Depression.
- Muscle weakness.
- Low blood pressure.
- Abnormal heartbeat.
- Heart attack.
- Facial flushing.
- Muscle weakness.
- Lethargy.
- Fatigue.
- Urine retention.

RDA:

- Adults: Males 350mg. Females: 320 mg.
- Pregnancy: 350 mg.
- Lactation: 320 mg.

Tolerable upper intake level:

- Adults: 350 mg.

87

"Nutritional supplementing with magnesium had a profound effect on my sleep!"

Steven Magee

<u>Zinc</u>

Zinc is widely used to boost immune system functioning. It is a common ingredient in cold and flu medications. You will also find it in hormone boosting supplements.

Function:

- Improves immune system.
- Zinc may shorten a cold.
- Lowers risk of pneumonia.
- Improves metabolism.
- Improves wound healing.
- Improves taste and smell.
- Prevents macular degeneration.
- Topical zinc oxide prevents diaper rash and sunburn.

Deficiency symptoms:

- Skin issues.
- Bone issues.
- Poor digestion.
- Diarrhea.
- Loss of appetite.
- Alopecia.
- Delayed growth.
- Affects reproductive system.

- Risk of child morbidity.
- Premature birth.
- Low birth weight.
- Affects central nervous system.
- Affects taste and smell.
- Delayed wound healing.
- Cognitive issues.
- Psychological issues.
- Affects immune system.
- Frequent infections.

Reported side effects:
- Indigestion.
- Diarrhea.
- Gastric distress.
- Loss of appetite.
- Nausea.
- Vomiting.
- Dizziness.
- Headaches.

Toxicity:
- May cause copper deficiency.
- Neurological issues.
- Sensory ataxia.
- Myelopathy.

- Anemia.

- Numbness and weakness in the arms and legs.

- Reduced immune function.

- Lower HDL cholesterol levels.

RDA:

- Adults: Males 11 mg. Females 8 mg.

Tolerable upper intake level:

- Infants under 6 months: 4 mg.

- Adults: 40 mg.

"The first few days of supplementing with a high dose of zinc brought on morning erections!"

Steven Magee

Alpha Lipoic Acid (ALA)

ALA is commonly used to detoxify the body. I could not tolerate it when I first took it and had to start on very low doses and gradually work my way up to high doses over several months. I regarded it to be an indication that my body had severe toxicity in it, as I had worked with many of the toxins it binds to.

Function:

- Antioxident.

- Enzymatic nutrient breakdown.

- Iron chelation.

- Binds to toxic metals (Fe, Zn, Hg, Pb, and Cu).

- Regenerates vitamin C.

- May reduce inflammation.

- Treats schemia-reperfusion injuries.

- Treats radiation injuries.

- May reduce diabetic neuropathy.

- May reduce metabolic syndrome.

- Stabilizes cognitive function.

- May slow cognitive decline.

Deficiency symptoms:

- Lipoic acid synthetase deficiency.

Reported side effects:

- Insomnia.

- Fatigue.

- Diarrhea.

- Skin rash.

- Allergic reaction: Hives; difficult breathing; swelling of your face, lips, tongue, or throat.

- Low blood sugar.

- Headache.

- Hunger.

- Weakness.

- Sweating.

- Confusion.

- Irritability.

- Dizziness.

- Fast heart rate.

- Feeling jittery.

- Light-headed.

- Feeling like you may pass out.

- Nausea.

Toxicity:

- Neurologic effects.

- May increase suicidal thoughts.

- May increase psychological issues.

- Tachycardia.

- Metabolic acidosis.

- T wave inversion in the EKG.

- Vomiting.

- Lethargy.

- Involuntary movements.

- Common in children.

RDA:

- Adults: 200 to 2400 mg.

Tolerable upper intake level:

- 2400 mg.

"My health significantly improved by taking alpha lipoic acid."

Steven Magee

<u>Amberen</u>

Amberen is marketed to females as a menopause relief supplement. My testing was indicating it works well in males also. The glycine it contains treats altitude hypersensitivity when taken in conjunction with L-Carnitine or L-Carnitine L-Tartrate.

Known health improvements:

- It may improve sleep.

- It may reduce stress.

- It may reduce night sweats.

- It may increase energy.

- Treats altitude hypersensitivity when taken with L-Carnitine.

Know side effects it may cause:

- Nausea.

- Headaches and migraine headaches.

- Constipation.

- Decreased energy.

- Bloating.

- Constipation.

- Fatigue.

- Limb pain.

Not suitable for:

- Those who are pregnant.

- Those who are breastfeeding.

- Those who have severe hypertension.

"Taking Amberen was how I discovered the treatment for Altitude Hypersensitivity."

Steven Magee

Testosterone Supplements

I had used "Weider Prime Testosterone Support" with success for a few years. It has the following ingredients in the 2 capsule serving:

- Vitamins:
  - D3 800 IU.
  - B6 10 mg.
  - B12 120 mcg.
- Calcium 35 mg.
- Zinc 15 mg.
- Chromium 200 mcg.
- Diindolymethane 50 mg.
- Asgwagandha extract 675 mg.
- Cordyceps extract 390 mg.
- Piperine 5 mg.

Regarding hypoxia, the supplement states that it improves cardio-respiratory endurance and improves oxygen consumption. At the recommended dose of two capsules daily, I found it was increasing daily fatigue.

As such, I dropped it back to one capsule daily and combined it with "Influx Inspire Extreme Test". It has the following ingredients in the 2 capsule serving:

- Proprietary Blend 1,484 mg containing:
  - Horny goat weed leaf extract.
  - Tongkat ali root extract.
  - Saw palmetto fruit extract.

- Orchic substance.
- Wild yam root extract.
- Sarsaparilla root extract.
- Nettle root extract.
- Boron amino acid chelate.

Of note, the boron amino acid chelate was believed to:

- Reduces the risk of lung cancer.

- Improves bone health.

- Reduces pain and inflammation.

- Reduces indicators of inflammation.

- Reduces yeast infections.

- Improves immune system.

- Increases the conversion of total testosterone in your body to free testosterone.

- Increases free testosterone.

- Reduces estradiol.

- Allows more free testosterone to bond with proteins in your blood.

- Builds muscles.

- Improves thinking.

Surprisingly, "Orchic Substance" is cows testicles! Yes, ground up cows testicles are believed to improve male health. Most of the ingredients listed are natural herbal remedies associated with improving health.

So I was taking one capsule of each in the morning daily. With the combined supplements I found that it caused the following side effects in the first week:

- Insomnia.

- Wide awake after midnight for an hour or so.

- Afternoon tiredness.

- Increased confusion.

As you can see, they were definitely causing the body to change. The side effects subsided after one week. After a week I was able to put it to the sex test. I had been taking:

- 45 days of Amberen.
  - One white capsule.
  - One orange capsule.
- 14 days of Weider Prime Testosterone Support.
  - One capsule.
- 7 days of Influx Inspire Extreme Test.
  - One capsule.

And I found it caused the following:

- Great sex.
- Daily sex at 1 to 2 times.
- Sexual stamina causing long lasting sex sessions.
- Sex testing lasted one week:
  - No loss of sexual desire or stamina was observed.
  - Achieving orgasm became difficult after several days as sperm production could not keep up with the rate of daily sex.

After the side effects passed through from adjusting to testosterone boosting supplements, I was very energized. Testing was so successful that I incorporated it into my daily supplement regimen. I really enjoyed researching this supplement combination!

It appears the supplements do offset the effects of "Descent Fatigue" from high altitude and it may be wise to take them prior to a mountain trip.

"Sometimes it is better to combine different formulations of supplements that claim to do the same thing."

Steven Magee

<u>Fish Oil Supplements</u>

Fish oils are commonly called omega 3 fatty acids. They are associated with good health and longevity.

Functions:

- Contains docosahexaenoic acid (DHA) and eicosapentaenoic acid (EPA).

- Reduces the risk of several chronic diseases.

- Reduces myocardial infarction.

- Reduces heart failure, coronary disease, and fatal coronary heart disease.

- Reduces arrhythmias.

- Reduces triglyceride levels.

- May lower blood pressure.

- Decreases platelet aggregation.

- Relieves inflammation.

- Reduces rates of all-cause mortality, cardiac death, sudden death, and stroke.

- Reduced risk of cognitive decline, Alzheimer's disease, and dementia.

- Lower risk of macular degeneration.

- May reduce high blood pressure.

- May reduce rheumatoid arthritis.

Deficiency symptoms:

- Rough, scaly skin.

- Dermatitis.

Reported side effects:

- Fishy aftertaste.

- Bad breath.

- Heartburn.

- Nausea.

- Diarrhea.

- Rash.

- Bleeding gums.

- Nosebleeds.

- Low blood pressure.

Toxicity:

- Increased blood sugar levels in people with diabetes.

- Vitamin A toxicity.

- Dizziness.

- Nausea.

- Joint pain.

- Skin irritation.

- Liver damage.

- Liver failure.

- Insomnia.

- May cause strokes.

RDA:

- Adults: 250–500 mg.

Tolerable upper intake level:

- 5,000 mg.

"Fish oil is known for its protective properties to human health."

Steven Magee

Live Culture Yogurt

Live culture plain yogurt is associated with better health and longevity. It colonizes the gastrointestinal tract with beneficial bacteria.

Functions:

- High in protein, calcium, vitamins, and live cultures.

- Enhances the gut microbiota.

- Probiotic foods may enhance absorption of vitamins and minerals.

- Aids digestion.

- Has lactic acid.

- Low lactose.

- Contains calcium, vitamins B6 and B12, riboflavin, potassium, and magnesium.

- Protection for bones and teeth.

- Contains natural hormones.

- May reduce digestive problems.

- May improve the immune system.

- Protects against osteoporosis.

- Reduces irritable bowel disease.

- May reduce type 2 diabetes.

- May help with weight loss.

- May reduce cardiovascular disease.

Side effects:

- Lactose intolerance.

- Milk allergy.

- Histamine problems.

- Acne.

- Eczema.

- May increase gastrointestinal problems.

- May cause gas.

- May cause bloating.

- May cause inflammatory issues.

- May cause weight gain.

"I eat a cup of natural plain yogurt with live cultures daily for good health."

Steven Magee

Amino Acids

Amino acids are commonly available and are marketed as sports supplements. They are proteins and are the basis of muscle growth. They also assist in workout recovery by detoxifying the body of ammonia that muscles produce in the blood. They are associated with energy production.

There are many health conditions that are treated by amino acids and they are called "Urea Cycle Disorders". They are common in children, as they are often genetic. The ratio of amino acids depends on the type of urea cycle disorder that is being treated.

There are hundreds of amino acids, although only 20 are regarded as needed by the human:

1. Alanine.

2. Arginine.

3. Asparagine.

4. Aspartate.

5. Cysteine.

6. Glutamine.

7. Glutamate.

8. Glycine.

9. Histidine.

10. Isoleucine.

11. Leucine.

12. Lysine.

13. Methionine.

14. Phenylalanine.

15. Proline.

16. Serine.

17. Threonine.

18. Tryptophan.

19. Tyrosine.

20. Valine.

Generally tryptophan is not seen in amino acid supplements, as it became linked to negative health issues in people that took it in 1989. It caused a large outbreak of eosinophilia-myalgia syndrome (EMS) from contaminated batches of supplements.

In the human diet, amino acids are mostly found in organ meats, such as the heart, liver and kidneys. It is notable that the organ meats have largely disappeared out of the human diet and will have reduced the amino acid levels of the modern human body. When was the last time you ate beef heart, deep fried beef lungs, steak and kidney pie or had liver and onions?

A single amino acid supplement can be problematic and may lead to a negative nitrogen balance. This can cause:

- Altered metabolism.

- Kidneys work harder.

When you see "L-" in front of an amino acid name, it means "Levorotatory". It indicates that it is easily absorbed into the body.

Essential amino acids are those that the body cannot make and have to be obtained from the diet. It is important that all of these essential amino acids are in your daily diet for good health. These are:

1. Valine.

2. Isoleucine.

3. Leucine.

4. Methionine.

5. Phenylalanine.

6. Tryptophan.

7. Threonine.

8. Histidine.

9. Lysine.

If one of the above amino acids is not consumed in the diet in sufficient quantities, then the body will have problems manufacturing proteins. A deficiency of one or more of the essential amino acids is described as "Protein-Energy Malnutrition".

There are others that are conditionally essential that the body has problems making when stressed:

1. Arginine.

2. Cysteine.

3. Glycine.

4. Glutamine.

5. Proline.

6. Tyrosine.

It is important that the above are taken during times of biological stress. Protein deficiency problems cause:

- Affects all organs.

- Affects many body systems.

- Affects brain development in infants and young children.

- Inhibits the immune system.

- Increased risk of infection.

- Affects gut mucosal function and permeability.

- Increases risks of systemic disease.

- Impacts kidney function.

- Edema.

- Failure to thrive in infants and children.

- Poor musculature.

- Dull skin.

- Thin and fragile hair.

- Low serum albumin.

- Low serum transferrin.

"High dosing of a single amino acid can be done for a short period of time, but long term it may cause issues."

Steven Magee

Essential Amino Energy

"Essential Amino Energy by Optimum Nutrition" was a supplement I had been testing for a few years. I could not really see much of an improvement in health on it when I lived at altitude in Tucson. When I moved out to Hawaii and was near sea level, the health improvement was noticeable. Amino acids have been a foundation of my pandemic supplements since I moved to Hawaii in 2021.

Amino energy has the following amino acids in it:

- Taurine.

- L-Glutamine.

- L-Arginine.

- L-Leucine.

- Beta-Alanine.

- L-Citrulline.

- L-Isoleucine.

- L-Valine.

- L-Tyrosine.

- L-Histidine.

- L-Lysine Hydrochloride.

- L-Phenylalanine.

- L-Threonine.

- L-Methionine.

The actual amounts are unknown, as it is listed as a 5 g "Amino Blend" and no individual quantities are given. It also has a 440 mg electrolyte blend of:

- Sodium Chloride.

- Magnesium Oxide.

- Potassium Chloride.

It is a stimulant based amino acid blend and it should only be taken in the mornings. It contains:

- Caffeine 100 mg.

- Green Tea Leaf Extract 50 mg.

- Green Coffee Bean Extract 10 mg.

It has a 4.7 out of 5 rating on amazon.com. I have used it a various daily doses from one scoop through to six scoops. I generally use it at the two scoop daily dose, which is one serving. It is a powder that is dissolved into water to make a drink. It tastes good! The manufacturer recommends it for:

- Pre-workout.

- During workout.

- Post workout.

- Anytime energy support.

- Focus.

- Hydration.

"The regular consumption of amino acids improved my health."

Steven Magee

Amino Acid Complex

"Amino Acid Complex by Horbaach" is a tablet based amino acid nutritional supplement. I use it for traveling, as it fits in a large pill box. It has the following amino acids in it:

- L-Alanine 255 mg.

- L-Arginine 261 mg.

- L-Aspartic Acid 168 mg.

- L-Glutamic Acid 336 mg.

- L-Glycine 618 mg.

- L-Histidine 42 mg.

- L-Hydroxylysine 12 mg.

- L-Hydroxyproline 333 mg.

- L-Isoleucine 42 mg.

- L-Leucine 96 mg.

- L-Lysine 106 mg.

- L-Methionine 27 mg.

- L-Phenylalanine 69 mg.

- L-Proline 414 mg.

- L-Serine 105 mg.

- L-Threonine 57 mg.

- L-Tyrosine 21 mg.

- L-Valine 69 mg.

It also contains:

- Vitamin C 30 mg.

- Sodium 30 mg.

From the above listing, you can see it is a very different nutritional supplement to essential amino energy! It is important to realize that amino acid nutritional supplements can be very different from each other.

It has a 4.5 out of 5 rating on amazon.com. For me, it appeared to be better than essential amino energy. I was very energized on this and it does not have stimulants in it!

It does have a large dose of L-Glycine in it, which I had identified as being part of the treatment for altitude hypersensitivity. Altitude hypersensitivity could probably be treated by combining this amino acid nutritional supplement with L-Carnitine. I have not tested this combination yet and cannot confirm if it works or not.

"I travel with amino acid tablets."

Steven Magee

<u>Glycine</u>

I first identified glycine as being import in my health through taking Amberen. Amberen treated the altitude hypersensitivity I had when taken with L-Carnitine. Further testing showed it was the glycine that Amberen contained that was treating altitude hypersensitivity. I have a deficiency that glycine treats and I always take glycine to treat it. Removing glycine from my nutritional supplements causes me to develop altitude hypersensitivity again.

Functions:

- Treats altitude hypersensitivity when taken with L-Carnitine.

- Anti-inflammatory.

- Lipid metabolization.

- Reduces platelets aggregation.

- Make proteins in the body.

- Involved in the transmission of chemical signals in the brain.

- Improves nerves.

- Production of serotonin.

- Component of collagen.

- Used to treat schizophrenia.

- Improves memory.

- Improves thinking.

- Improves mood.

- Treats stroke.

- Treats heart disease.
- May help with ischemia-reperfusion injury.
- Protects against narrowing of the arteries.
- May help protect the liver from toxins.
- Treats insomnia.
- Treats benign prostatic hyperplasia (BPH).
- Treats metabolic disorders.
- Treats leg ulcers.
- Treats diabetes.
- Believed to prevent cancer.
- Removes toxins from the body.

Deficiency symptoms:

- Arginine glycine amidinotransferase deficiency.
- Mild to moderate intellectual disability.
- Delayed speech development.
- Autistic behaviors.
- Affects communication.
- Affects social interaction.
- Seizures.
- Failure for children to thrive.
- Delayed development of motor skills.
- Weak muscle tone.
- Tire easily.

Reported side effects:

- Nausea.
- Vomiting.
- Stomach upset.
- Diarrhea.
- Drowsiness.

Toxicity:

- Avoid use during pregnancy or lactation.
- Avoid use in children.
- Glycine encephalopathy.
- Visual disturbances.
- Drowsiness.
- Vomiting.
- Weakness.
- Prickling skin sensations.
- Skin flushing.
- Can be fatal.

RDA:

- 2 to 5 g.

Tolerable upper intake level:

- Adult: 6 g.

"Glycine significantly improved my health!"

Steven Magee

L-Carnitine

L-Carnitine became a key component of my research into altitude hypersensitivity. I had been testing the nutritional supplement and I noticed altitude hypersensitivity subsided when taking it. I was able to link it to glycine. Taking both of them together prevents altitude hypersensitivity from occurring.

Function:

- Prevents altitude hypersensitivity when combined with glycine.

- Body can produce L-Carnitine from lysine and methionine.

- Critical for mitochondrial fatty acid β-oxidation.

- Treatment of primary systemic carnitine deficiency, propionyl-CoA carboxylase deficiency and medium chain acyl-CoA dehydrogenase deficiency.

- Treats cardiovascular disease.

- May reduce peripheral neuropathy.

- May reduce depression.

- May reduce Alzheimer's disease.

- May reduce hepatic encephalopathy.

- May help with weight loss.

Deficiency symptoms:

- Primary systemic carnitine deficiency.

- Hypoketotic hypoglycemia.

- Encephalopathy.

- Hepatomegaly.

- Elevated liver enzymes.

- Hypoammonemia in infants.

- Progressive cardiomyopathy.

- Elevated creatine kinase.

- Skeletal myopathy in childhood.

- Fatigability in adulthood.

- Secondary carnitine deficiency.

- Buildup of organic acids.

- Fanconi's syndrome.

- Abnormal profiles of acylcarnitine esters in blood.

Reported side effects:

- Nausea.

- Vomiting.

- Abdominal cramps.

- Diarrhea.

- Fishy body odor.

RDA:

- Adults: 0.5 to 2 g

Tolerable upper intake level:

- No upper limit has been established.

"L-Carnitine is associated with good heart health."

Steven Magee

L-Carnitine L-Tartrate

I had to use L-Carnitine L-Tartrate during the COVID -19 pandemic because supply shortages had caused L-Carnitine to go out of stock. L-Carnitine L-Tartrate works with glycine to prevent altitude hypersensitivity from occurring.

Function:

- Works with glycine to prevent altitude hypersensitivity.
- Chemoprotective.
- Antioxidant.
- L-Tartrate is a potent antioxidant.
- Increases fatty acid oxidation.
- Reduces purine catabolism.
- Reduces free radical formation.
- Involved in ATP production.
- May prevent exercise fatigue.
- Reduces muscle weakness.
- Reduces peripheral neuropathy.
- Reduces hyperlipoproteinemia.

Deficiency symptoms:

- Comparable to L-Carnitine deficiency.

Reported side effects:

- Dry mouth.

- Upset stomach.
- Heartburn.
- Nausea.
- Vomiting.
- Diarrhea.
- Abdominal cramps.
- Loss of appetite.
- Weight loss.
- Headache.
- Muscle pain.
- Muscle weakness.
- Swelling of hands, lower legs or feet.
- Tingling skin.
- Fishy body odor.
- Hypertension
- Arrhythmias.
- Chest pain or angina.
- Electrocardiogram irregularities.
- Palpitations.
- Vascular disorder.
- Seizures
- Hypertonia.
- Insomnia.
- Paresthesia.
- Vertigo.

- Headache.

- Restlessness.

- Hypercalcemia.

- Hyperkalemia.

- Hypervolemia.

RDA:

- Adults: 1 to 4 g.

Tolerable upper intake level:

- Unknown.

"L-Carnitine L-Tartrate is linked to improved outcomes in COVID-19 infections."

Steven Magee

GPLC

My testing with supplements that treated altitude hypersensitivity was indicating that it may be the combination of L-Carnitine and glycine that were the actual treatment. Research revealed such a supplement existed and it was called GPLC. Two types of GPLC were obtained and tested and both treated altitude hypersensitivity. This confirmed the combination of L-Carnitine and glycine were the actual supplements required for the treatment.

Functions:

- Antioxidant.

- Supports testosterone.

- Supports growth hormone.

- Supports nitric oxide.

- Improves insulin resistance.

- May assist in weight loss.

- May improve energy.

- Reduces oxidative stress.

- Heart protective.

- Improves erectile dysfunction.

Deficiency symptoms:

- May cause altitude hypersensitivity.

Reported side effects:

- Nausea.

- Diarrhea.

- Appetite.

- Sleeplessness.

- Increased body odor.

RDA:

- Adults: 1 to 4.5g.

Tolerable upper intake level:

- Unknown.

"GPLC is the only nutritional supplement I know of that will treat Altitude Hypersensitivity on its own."

Steven Magee

L-Arginine

L-Arginine improved sexual functioning in me. I associate it with long lasting sex sessions.

Functions:

- Precursor to nitric oxide, polyamines, proline, glutamate, creatine, citrulline and agmatine.

- Improves athletic performance.

- Helps build proteins.

- Builds muscles.

- Wound healing.

- Treats heart conditions.

- Treats Angina.

- Treats high blood pressure.

- Treats erectile dysfunction.

- Treats preeclampsia.

- Treats peripheral arterial disease.

- Treats migraines.

Deficiency symptoms:

- Arginase deficiency (Argininemia).

- Hyperammonemia.

- Children have slow growth, developmental delays and cognitive problems.

- Brain lesions.

- Liver damage.

- T cell dysfunction.

- Endothelial dysfunction.

- Disrupts many cellular and organ functions.

Reported side effects:

- Dizziness.

- Gastrointestinal issues.

- Nausea.

- Vomiting.

- Abdominal pain.

- Diarrhea.

- Bloating.

- Gout.

- Headache.

- Allergic response.

- Airway inflammation.

- Worsening of asthma symptoms.

- Difficulty breathing or a tight feeling in your chest.

Toxicity:

- Not for use in recent heart attacks, as it may increase risk of death.

- Heart failure.

- May worsen allergies or asthma.

- Too much may trigger cold sores or genital herpes.

- May cause low blood pressure.

- May lower blood sugar levels.

- Not recommended for pregnancy or lactation.

- May cause tumor growth.

RDA:

- Adults: 2 to 30 g.

Tolerable upper intake level:

- Adults: 30 g.

"*L-Arginine has the potential to improve your relationship!*"
Steven Magee

L-Citrulline

L-Citrulline caused a major improvement in health for me. I started to feel more normal the longer I took it.

Functions:

- Antioxidant.

- Body converts it to arginine.

- Increases arginine levels.

- Boosts nitric oxide production.

- May improve athletic performance.

- May decrease muscle soreness.

- May lower blood pressure.

- Improves wound healing.

- Treats erectile dysfunction.

- Treats short bowel syndrome.

- Treats celiac disease.

- Treats radiation induced small bowel damage.

- Treats liver disease.

- Improves Parkinson's disease.

- Improves dementia.

Deficiency symptoms:

- Citrullinemia.

- Infants:

- - Vomiting.
  - Refusal to eat.
  - Lethargy.
  - Intracranial pressure.
  - Seizures.
  - Loss of consciousness.
- Neurologic deficits.
- Hyperammonemia.
- Body becomes toxic.
- Liver problems.
- Intense headaches.
- Blind spots.
- Balance issues.
- Muscle coordination issues.
- Lethargy.
- Affects nervous system.
- Confusion.
- Restlessness.
- Memory loss.
- Abnormal behaviors.
- Aggression.
- Irritability.
- Hyperactivity.
- Seizures
- Coma.
- Avoidance of carbohydrates.

- Can be life-threatening.

- Can be triggered by certain medications, infections, surgery, and alcohol intake.

- Neonatal intrahepatic cholestasis caused by citrin deficiency (NICCD).
  - Failure to thrive.
  - Dyslipidemia.
  - Delayed growth.
  - Extreme tiredness.
  - Fatigue.
  - Abnormal amounts of fats (lipids) in the blood (dyslipidemia).

Reported side effects:

- Gastrointestinal upset.

- Bloating.

- Cramping.

- Diarrhea.

- Sweating.

Toxicity:

- Unknown.

RDA:

- 3 to 6 g.

Tolerable upper intake level:

- 6 g.

"L-Citrulline really boosted my health!"

Steven Magee

L-Lysine

L-Lysine was used to treat my suspected protein intolerance. I felt better after adding it into my daily nutritional supplements.

Functions:

- Aids absorption of calcium, iron, and zinc.
- Used to produce enzymes, antibodies, and hormones.
- Supports immune system.
- Supports cell function.
- May reduce anxiety.
- May prevent cold sores.
- Improves calcium absorption.
- Reduces cortisol levels.
- Promotes wound healing.
- Essential for the formation of collagen.
- Treats schizophrenia.
- May reduce blood pressure.
- May prevent cancer.
- May aid blood sugar levels.

Deficiency symptoms:

- Loss of appetite.
- Broken skin.

- Fragile nails.
- Dizziness.
- Fatigue.
- Anemia.
- Mood changes.
- Poor concentration.
- Irritability.
- Nausea.
- Red eyes.
- Hair loss.
- Anorexia.
- Inhibited growth.
- Problems with the reproductive system.

Reported side effects:
- Diarrhea.
- Nausea.
- Stomach cramps.

Toxicity:
- Children should avoid it.
- Not recommended for pregnancy or lactation.
- Kidney problems.
- Gallstones.
- Higher cholesterol.
- Should be avoided by people with kidney or liver issues.

RDA:

- Adults: 1 to 3 g.

Tolerable upper intake level:

- Unknown.

"L-Lysine is an essential amino acid that may prevent cold sores."

Steven Magee

<u>Creatine</u>

Creatine came to my attention for its use for treating the "Hypoxia Blues" that is known to occur in people living at high altitudes.

Function:

- Made from three amino acids: glycine, arginine, and methionine.

- Treats altitude sickness.

- Increases muscle size, strength and power.

- Improves athletic performance.

- Improves brain functioning.

- Prevents muscle cramps.

- Reduces fatigue.

- Improves multiple sclerosis.

- Treats depression.

Deficiency symptoms:

- Creatine deficiency disorders:
  - Creatine biosynthesis disorders guanidinoacetate methyltransferase (GAMT) deficiency.
  - L-arginine:glycine amidinotransferase (AGAT) deficiency.
  - Creatine transporter (CRTR) deficiency.

- Developmental delay.

- Cognitive dysfunction.

- Intellectual disability.

- Speech-language disorder.

- Epilepsy.

- Behavioral disorders.

- Hyperactivity.

- Autism.

- Self injury.

- Movement disorder.

- Attention deficit.

- Impulsivity.

- Social anxiety.

- Aggressive behavior.

- Hypotonia.

- Poor weight gain.

- Constipation.

- Prolonged QTc on EKG.

- Severe intellectual disability in adults.

Reported side effects:

- Weight gain.

- Bloating.

- Diarrhea.

- Stomach upset.

- Belching.

Toxicity:

- May harm kidneys.

- Not recommended for kidney disease.

RDA:

- Adults: 3 to 5 g.

Tolerable upper intake level:

- Adults: Unknown.

"Doctors have been treating altitude sickness induced depression with creatine for many years."

Steven Magee

Digestive Enzymes

Digestive enzymes can help with nutrition absorption into the body. They help to create the correct environment in the digestive tract to assist with the absorption of food and nutritional supplements. If you have issues with digestion, they can help increase the nutritional status of the body.

During my research, I have used the following digestive enzyme supplements:

- NOW Super Enzymes.
  - Rated 4.6 out of 5.
- Revly Digestive Enzyme Complex.
  - Rated 4.3 out of 5.
- Doctor's Best Betaine HCI Pepsin & Gentian Bitters.
  - Rated 4.5 out of 5.
- Zenwise Digestive Enzymes.
  - Rated 4.4 out of 5.

A digestive enzyme is taken every time something is eaten. They will help break down the food for absorption into the body.

I have gone on and off digestive enzymes over the years. I generally will start taking them if I think something is up with my digestion that they can fix. If I see no results, I stop taking them.

They appear to be particularly useful to those with a damaged intestinal tract that may have lost part of it due to surgery.

The digestive enzyme I use today is yogurt with live cultures.

"Digestive enzymes can help offset nutrient absorption problems in the digestive tract."

Steven Magee

Colon Cleanse

The gastrointestinal system is greatly affected by COVID - 19. Gastrointestinal problems are one of the most commonly reported symptoms of COVID-19. Long COVID patients are showing traces of the COVID-19 virus in their stools a year after the initial infection!

I became interested in organ cleanses due to hearing stories of people that had improved their health with them. Various cleanses exist for the organs and have highly rated reviews on amazon.com. Most people have a level of toxicity in their organs from modern life. These organ cleanses assist with reducing that toxicity.

The top one to do is the colon cleanse. The colon is filled with lots of fungus, bacteria, viruses and parasites and they accumulate with time. "Irritable Bowl Syndrome" is a common diagnosis in modern society and colon cancer is rapidly rising in the global population. The foundation of good health is a healthy colon!

The gastrointestinal system is often called the "Second Brain" because it is strongly linked to brain functioning. A poorly functioning colon may induce a myriad of brain functioning issues into you! Once the chemical balance is off in the colon, it will likely stay off until a colon cleanse or a long term fast is performed.

During my time passing through gastrointestinal departments in Tucson, I was never told to cleanse the colon. I was never prescribed a colon cleanse. The closest thing to it I received was the preparation for a colonoscopy. For that, you starve yourself for 24 hours while drinking a laxative solution that cleans the colon. Then you have your colonoscopy and start eating normally afterwards.

I was smart enough to know that the colonoscopy procedure destroys the flora of the gastrointestinal tract and it was unwise to eat normally after it. I knew reintroducing known good probiotics was important after having this procedure done. This would recolonize the colon from the outset with good bacteria. I took a variety of probiotics during the months after the procedure and ate a very clean organic diet. My gastrointestinal symptoms were greatly reduced afterwards, although I was still food intolerant. The gastroenterologists could not tell me why I was food intolerant and could not fix the food intolerance. I tested negative for "Celiac Disease", even though I was gluten intolerant.

I have used the following colon cleanses in the years afterwards:

- Dr. Tobias Colon 14 Day Cleanse.

    - Rated 4.3 stars out of 5.

- Advanced 15 Day Colon Detox and Cleanse by Bio Schwartz.

    - Rated 3.9 stars out of 5.

Colon cleansing changes the gastrointestinal tract flora and it is normal to feel a bit weird and experience unusual health symptoms during the cleanse. Afterward I have always felt better! It is something I regularly do once per year now.

"It is important to do annual maintenance on the gastrointestinal tract."

Steven Magee

Kidney Cleanse

Kidney issues have been widely reported in COVID-19 infections and Long COVID survivors. The stress of the infection and the hypoxia it causes are known to damage the organs, including the kidneys. The kidneys are regarded as one of the most sensitive organs to low blood oxygen levels and are easily damaged by it.

Similar to the colon cleanse, the kidney cleanse will help detoxify the kidneys. I have used:

- Dr. Bo Kidney Cleanse.
  - Rated 4.4 stars out of 5.

It does cause a change in health during the cleanse and I did feel different while taking it. Afterwards I felt better! Given that I appear to have kidney issues that are causing amino acid problems in the body, I now do a regular annual kidney cleanse to help my kidneys detoxify.

"I am medically trained in kidney dialysis."

Steven Magee

Liver Cleanse

Severe cases of COVID-19 are known to damage the liver. The damage is associated with lung lesions which presumably cause hypoxia to occur in the liver. The liver is an organ that is known to be damaged by hypoxia.

I have used these liver cleanses:

- Lifestyle Awareness Dandy Liver Detox Tea.
  - Rated 4.6 stars out of 5.
- Dr. Tobias Liver 21 Day Cleanse.
  - Rated 4.2 stars out of 5.

I also will be testing out these ones in the near future:

- Envy Nutrition Liver Cleanse.
  - Rated 4.3 stars out of 5.
- Vimerson Health Liver Health.
  - Rated 4.3 stars out of 5.

I generally have noticed changed health during the liver cleanses and improved health afterwards. I do consider regular colon, kidney and liver cleanses as a foundation of good health. It is well known that organ functioning degrades with age. It is a good idea to give them a tune up from time to time.

"Cherry Angiomas" (Liver Spots) on your skin are a sign that liver damage may be present.

"I have had red liver spots on my skin for many years now."

Steven Magee

Monster Energy Drink

I have an extensive history with green "Monster Energy" drinks. When I first started to experience chronic fatigue during hypoxic extreme night shift work atop the 13,800 feet high Mauna Kea volcano in Hawaii, USA, I was drinking a lot of it! It is similar to another energy drink called "Red Bull" which I was also drinking to try and stay awake during the daytime. They initially worked, but long term use rendered them ineffective and I would drink them and go to sleep anyway! I had become tolerant to them and the underlying health conditions I was trying to treat with them were progressing. It was the start of my long term struggle with chronic fatigue.

Monster energy came back onto my RADAR in 2023 when I was given a free can with a purchase. At the time I had been experiencing headaches for days as I was trying to develop the third pandemic supplement protocol. I was changing my nutritional supplement intake at the time and the assumption was the headaches were coming out of a nutritional deficiency I had.

I like the taste of monster energy and I drank it with my morning supplements. That day the headaches cleared up and I have never seen them since! It only required one can of the drink to clear them up. So what is in monster energy? It has the following:

- Riboflavin (B2) 260%.

- Niacin (B3) 250%.

- Vitamin B6 240%.

- Vitamin B12 500%.

- Glucose.

- Taurine.

- Panax ginger extract.

- L-Carnitine.

- Caffeine.

- Glucuronolactone.

- Inositol.

- Gurana extract.

- Maltodextrin.

As you can see from the above, it is a nutritional health drink. Adding it to my nutritional intake for one day cleared up the headaches! So something on the above list cleared them up and I have no idea what it was!

"Many discoveries are accidental!"

Steven Magee

<u>Coffee</u>

Many people with chronic fatigue drink coffee. It does help and I am a regular coffee drinker because of it. I do not need coffee today, but do continue to drink it.

Function:

- Antioxidant.

- Contains caffeine.

- Source of vitamin B2 (riboflavin).

- Source of Magnesium.

- Has plant chemicals: polyphenols including chlorogenic acid and quinic acid, and diterpenes including cafestol and kahweol.

- Increased alertness.

- Increased energy.

- Improves concentration.

- Improves mood.

- May reduce risk of colorectal cancer.

- May prevent or reduce Parkinson's disease.

- May reduce dementia.

- May reduce the risk of gallstones.

- May reduce the risk of developing diabetes.

- May reduce heart attack risks.

- May reduce risk of stroke.

- May reduce liver disease.

- May reduce obesity.

Reported side effects:

- Insomnia.

- Nervousness.

- Restlessness.

- Stomach upset.

- Nausea.

- Vomiting.

- Increased heart rate.

- Increased breathing rate.

- Pregnancy:
  - Increased risk of miscarriage.
  - Increased risk of premature birth.
  - Increased risk of low birth weight.

- Lactation:
  - May irritate infant digestive tract.
  - May cause infant sleep problems.
  - May cause infant irritability.

Toxicity:

- Anxiety.

- Agitation.

- Restlessness.

- Headache.

- Ringing in the ears.

- Irregular heartbeats.

- Diarrhea.

- May cause osteoporosis.

- Unfiltered coffee:
    - Increases total cholesterol.
    - Increases low-density lipoprotein (LDL).
    - Increases triglycerides.
    - May increase the risk of heart disease.

RDA:

- Adults: 1 to 5 cups.

Tolerable upper intake level:

- Adults: 5 cups.

"I have been a regular coffee drinker since I was twenty-six years old."

Steven Magee

Pandemic Supplements 1

This was the first supplementation system I developed for treating altitude hypersensitivity. Its secondary purpose was to treat lysinuric protein intolerance:

Steven Magee takes daily:

- Daily multivitamin.
  - Kirkland Signature.
- Calcium citrate, magnesium and zinc.
  - Kirkland Signature.
- Wild alaskan salmon oil 1,000 mg.
  - Pure Alaska Omega.
- Betaine HCI, pepsin and genetian bitters.
  - Doctor's best.
- Vitamin B12 5,000 mcg.
  - Kirkland Signature.
- Vitamin C 1,000 mg.
  - Kirkland Signature.
- Vitamin D 10,000 IU.
  - Carlyle.
- Alpha Lipoic Acid 300 mg.
  - Puritan's Pride.
- Folic acid 400 mcg.
  - Sundown.
- Iron 65 mg.

- ○ Nature Made.
- Creatine Monohydrate 3 g.
  - ○ Now Sports.
- Amino acid drink 10 g.
  - ○ Essential amino energy by Optimum Nutrition.
- L-Citrulline 6 g.
  - ○ Bulk Supplements.
- L-Lysine-HCL 1.5 g.
  - ○ Bulk Supplements.
- Acetyl-L-Carnitine HCl 750 mg.
  - ○ Jacked Factory.
- L-Arginine 500 mg.
  - ○ Jacked Factory.
- Amberen.
  - ○ Biogix, Inc.
- Testosterone Support one capsule.
  - ○ Weider Prime.
- Extreme Test one capsule.
  - ○ Influx Inspire.
- Breakfast is a pot of coffee (12 cups - 60 ounces) slowly consumed between sunrise and noon.
  - ○ Kirkland Signature whole bean french roast coffee.
  - ○ Kirkland Signature organic coffee creamer french vanilla flavored.

The iron tablet can be replaced with an iron fish, which may be more effective in the long term. "Kirkland" branded products are obtained at Costco.

The supplements are taken at breakfast, around 7 am. Missing a dose of the supplements generally causes sleepiness and fatigue to occur by 3 pm onward. This can be offset by taking the missed supplements. If the missed supplements are not taken until the next morning, then a progressive feeling of sickness will occur during the night. Taking the supplements the next morning clears the sickness.

Regarding food intake, I only drink liquids in the morning until noon. Breakfast is coffee and creamer. Lunch and dinner are solids and they are eaten between noon and 6pm. Food and drink intake is as follows:

- Sunrise: Wake up and spend 30 minutes outdoors.

- Morning: Take supplements with coffee and creamer.

- Noon: Start eating solids for lunch.

- 5pm: Solids dinner.

- 6pm: Start fasting, drink water only if needed.

- Sunset: Watch sunset for light absorption into the body to prepare it for sleep.

- Once the onset of tiredness takes place, go to bed with the curtains open for starlight, planet and moonlight exposures during sleep. The head of the bed needs to be under the window so that nighttime light can shine onto the face.

- Food fasting starts at 6pm and goes through to sunrise the next day.

- Liquids fast is typically 12 hours long.

- Liquids are only consumed for approximately 12 hours per day.

- Solids fast is typically 18 hours long.

- Solids are only eaten for 6 hours per day.

The supplements need to be taken in conjunction with daily outdoor exercise. That exercise should be a mix of cardio and muscle building exercise that is done for at least an hour. Vigorous swimming, lifting weights and/or cycling hills are effective. Regular sex is an excellent cardio exercise.

Long term testing over several months revealed the side effects of this supplement plan:

- Nerve damage at 9,200 feet occurred after an altitude test. (May not be related to the supplements.)

- Sore knees.

- Cramping in the right foot and right hand.

Sleeping blood oxygen was good for me at 93.8% average SpO2 and 60.8 average BPM pulse rate. The following graph shows the results.

"Nutritional supplements had far more beneficial effects than any of the prescription drugs."

Steven Magee

Pandemic Supplements 1 Sleeping SpO2 Graph

Blood oxygen during sleep was relatively stable and averaged 93.8% SpO2.

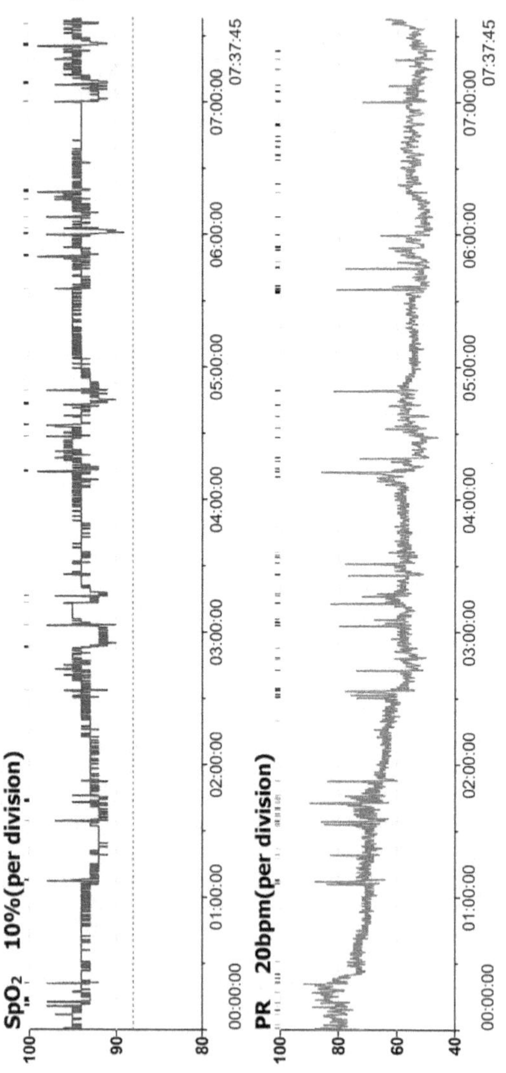

Minimum Supplements

One of the things I like to do is find out what are the minimum amount of supplements I need to take to maintain improved health. As such, I removed some of supplements I thought were non-essential at the time to see if I would continue in good health. The following were removed in August 2022:

- Daily multivitamin.
  - Kirkland Signature.
- Wild alaskan salmon oil 1,000 mg.
  - Pure Alaska Omega.
- Betaine HCI, pepsin and genetian bitters.
  - Doctor's best.
- Creatine Monohydrate 3 g.
  - Now Sports.
- Acetyl-L-Carnitine HCI 750 mg.
  - Jacked Factory.
- L-Arginine 500 mg.
  - Jacked Factory.

I did see an adverse reaction to removing Creatine Monohydrate. It caused severe sensitivity in my teeth, it was so severe that I could only eat liquid foods after five days of not taking it. The sensitive teeth subsided after two weeks. Stopping Acetyl-L-Carnitine HCI did bring on sensitive teeth for a couple of days.

The reduced supplements did have a negative effect on sexual functioning and reintroducing the full range of supplements fixed it. I had better sex and sexual stamina on the full range of supplements.

"It is important to experiment with supplements to verify you actually need to take them. Taking a non-essential supplement is just wasting your money."

Steven Magee

Pandemic Supplements 2

This supplement plan was developed to eliminate the knee pains that the first one was causing. It was suspected the knee pains were coming from supplement toxicity, so known toxic supplements were removed. Some supplements that were thought not to be needed anymore were also removed. The removed supplements did clear up the knee pains.

Steven Magee takes daily:

- Daily multivitamin.
  - Kirkland Signature.
- Calcium citrate, magnesium and zinc.
  - Kirkland Signature.
- Wild alaskan salmon oil 1,000 mg.
  - Pure Alaska Omega.
- Vitamin C 1,000 mg.
  - Kirkland Signature.
- Amino acid drink 10 g.
  - Essential amino energy by Optimum Nutrition.
- L-Citrulline 6 g.
  - Bulk Supplements.
- L-Lysine-HCL 1.5 g.
  - Bulk Supplements.
- Acetyl-L-Carnitine HCI 750 mg.
  - Jacked Factory.
- L-Arginine 500 mg.

- - Jacked Factory.

- Amberen.
  - Biogix, Inc.

- Testosterone Support one capsule.
  - Weider Prime.

- Extreme Test one capsule.
  - Influx Inspire.

- Breakfast is a pot of coffee (12 cups - 60 ounces) slowly consumed between sunrise and noon.
  - Kirkland Signature whole bean french roast coffee.
  - Kirkland Signature organic coffee creamer french vanilla flavored.

- Kidney Cleanse as needed.
  - Dr. Bo.

Sexual performance was excellent with long lasting sex sessions. It was further improved by doubling the dose of the testosterone boosting supplements.

A kidney cleanse was performed during this supplement protocol due to recognizing that the kidneys were involved in the amino acid deficiencies I have.

Sleeping blood oxygen was good for me at 94% average SpO2 and 51.7 average BPM pulse rate. The following graph shows the results. It was taken after a daytime exposure to driving at 2,000 feet and near sea level in Kona. Sleeping spikes into lower blood oxygen were a feature of pandemic supplement protocol 2.

"It is important to know which supplements you are taking are associated with toxicity to the human."

Steven Magee

159

"It is important to know which supplements you are taking are associated with toxicity to the human."

Steven Magee

Pandemic Supplements 2 Sleeping SpO2 Graph

Blood oxygen during sleep was relatively stable and averaged 94% SpO2.

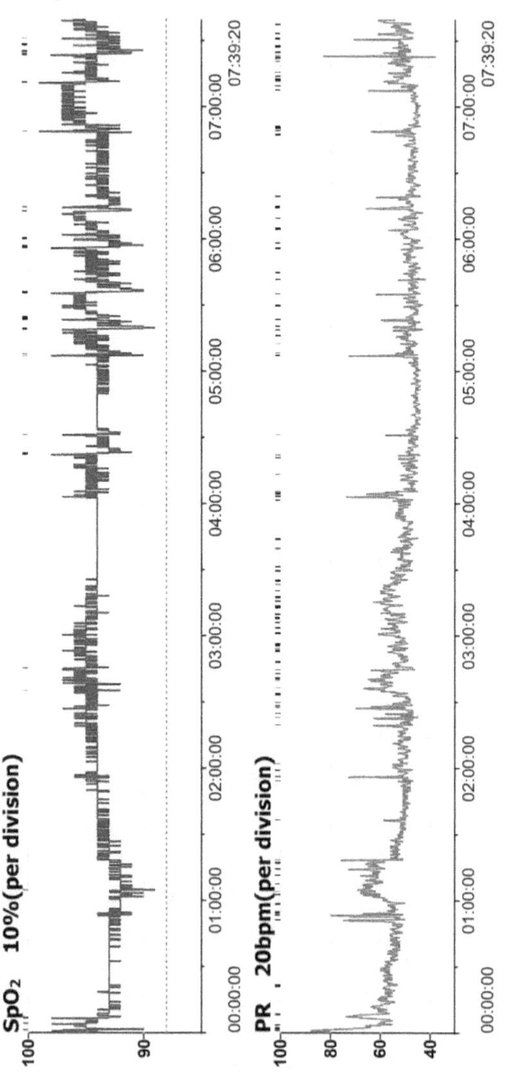

Pandemic Supplements 3

This set of supplements was for improved nail and skin growth. I was still having fungal toe nail growth and I was suspicious the fungal infection was systemic. I had a history of skin tags on my body after my flu-like illness in 2015. Research indicated the most effective treatment for fungal nails was an oral anti-fungal medication. This set of supplements was developed to attempt to counteract a systemic fungal infection.

The Amberen and L-Carnitine were removed, as I wanted to see if they could be replaced by GPLC to treat altitude hypersensitivity. Testing went well with GPLC and it does effectively treat altitude hypersensitivity.

The amino acid powders were removed to make it easier to travel. Traveling through airports with white powdered amino acids may flag you up to TSA as a suspected drugs dealer. I have had this experience in Kona airport in Hawaii and it is unpleasant! They tested all of the powders for drugs and it delayed me going through TSA! It was all done in front of the passengers going through the TSA area, so the passengers know what is going on. I got some strange looks from passengers once I was inside the airport gate area!

Two weeks after the amino acid powders were removed, the food sensitivities came back. I was getting very sleepy after some large evening meals. I introduced a 1,000 mg tablet of L-Arginine daily and within a few days, the food sensitivities were reduced but not completely gone. Adding Citrulline to it brought on headaches but did not clear up the food sensitivities. I happened to drink a can of "Monster Energy" with my morning supplements that I had got free with a purchase at a store. This completely cleared the headaches up!

Why would "Monster Energy" clear up the headaches? It has some extra supplements in it that were not in my regular daily supplements:

- Taurine.

- Panax Ginseng.

- L-Carnitine L-Tartrate.

- Guarana.

- Other ingredients.

There is something in this drink that interacted with my supplements to clear up the headaches. It required just one 16 fluid ounces can to be taken with the morning supplements. I suspect the "Monster Energy" was acting as a catalyst that increased or altered the pre-existing chemistry of my supplements. It triggered a beneficial reaction that only required one dose. Once the reaction had occurred, my existing supplements were sufficient at preventing headaches and they did not return. The ingredients in "Monster Energy" has commonality with some of the supplements that were used in the pandemic supplement protocols described in this book.

Food intolerance was still present in the evening after eating a large evening meal, bringing on tiredness and sleepiness. Mental functioning was beginning to decline and I was starting to feel weird brain functioning. It seemed the travel supplements were not fully treating the nutritional deficiencies I had.

The home where I was staying had a canister of "Amino Energy" and decided to start taking the full recommended dose of six scoops daily. I would take two scoops as soon as I woke up, another two scoops mid-morning and the final two scoops at lunchtime. This cleared up the food intolerance and brain functioning issues after one week.

Adjusting to six scoops daily of "Amino Energy" did bring on the following conditions in the first week:

- Nerve pains.

- Dreams.

Once the adjustment took place, the symptoms subsided and I was feeling good again! Lots of energy daily, no fatigue and good mental functioning.

The "Amino Energy" powder was replaced with amino acid tablets called "Amino Acid Complex 3000mg" by Horbaach. There was a mild headache reaction after several days that lasted for a day and cleared with sleep. I did get a brief period where I could remember dreaming for a few days. I remained free of symptoms and had developed a tablet based amino acid supplementation protocol that worked for me.

I stopped taking the multivitamin and replaced it with B-complex. This was due to being on the multivitamin for almost a year and I wanted to take a break from it.

I decided to replace the calcium citrate, magnesium and zinc with just magnesium and to increase the dose. This was due to seeing an increase in sleeping oxygen events.   I took the magnesium up to 250 mg from 80 mg daily.

The supplement system did not feel quite right, so a little research on it revealed it was very similar to what is being used to treat autistic children. Zinc is a big feature of that treatment. As such, I raised the zinc levels by adding a 50 mg zinc tablet daily. The reviews of the zinc supplement were showing 50 mg daily was well tolerated by most people.

Memory and confusion had slowly increased during developing this supplement protocol and had subsided once it had been fully developed.

The increased levels of the amino acids in the prior supplement protocols appear to improve sexual functioning. Adding in the zinc brought on morning erections and improved things. Sexual functioning waned during development of this supplement protocol before normalizing once completed.

Steven Magee takes daily:
- Magnesium Citrate 250 mg.

- Nature Made.
- Zinc 50 mg.
  - Nature's Bounty.
- Wild alaskan salmon oil 1,000 mg.
  - Pure Alaska Omega.
- Super B complex with vitamin C one tablet.
  - CVS Health.
- Vitamin C 2,000 mg.
  - Kirkland Signature.
- Vitamin E 180 mg.
  - Kirkland Signature.
  - For external use. Paint one capsule onto affected fungal nails and skin daily after showering.
- Vitamin E 1,440 mg.
  - Kirkland Signature.
- Biotin 10,000 mcg.
  - Bronson.
- GPLC two capsules.
  - Carlyle.
- L-Arginine & L-Citrulline one tablet.
  - Amazing Nutrition.
- Amino Acid Complex three tablets.
  - Horbaach.
- Testosterone Support one capsule.
  - Weider Prime.
- Extreme Test one capsule.
  - Influx Inspire.

- Organic greek yogurt plain one tablespoon with each meal.
  - Kirkland.
- Breakfast is a pot of coffee (12 cups - 60 ounces) slowly consumed between sunrise and noon.
  - Kirkland Signature whole bean french roast coffee.
  - Full cream milk.
- "Monster Energy" 16 fluid ounces if needed.
  - Monster Energy Company.

Sore shoulders and neck were observed in the first few weeks of taking this supplement combination and it slowly subsided. It was suspected to be the adjustment to the high dose of vitamin E. The area of my upper back and neck soreness were consistent with the area associated with Kyphosis. Kyphosis is an abnormally excessive convex curvature of the spine as it occurs in the thoracic and sacral regions.

Stools were looser on this supplement protocol and it was thought to be the anti-fungal properties of vitamin E that were affecting the contents of the digestive tract. Daily morning defecations were easy and pleasant.

Improved nail and hair growth was observed during the time I have been taking this supplement protocol. I expect to take it for at least six months to maintain the anti-fungal levels in the body. At the time of publication, I was three months into the high dosing of vitamin E and was not noticing any side effects or toxicity associated with it.

I was free of food intolerance symptoms and could eat a normal diet. I was not avoiding any food types. I could eat a huge pepperoni pizza from Costco without any issues.

This supplement system produced the highest energy levels. I was very alert and capable on it. A lot of jobs were getting done on my home!

After I wrapped up research on pandemic supplements 3, my supply of GPLC ran out. I noticed glycine was contained within the amino acid complex tablets and all I had to do was add in the L-Carnitine to replace the GPLC. I had L-Carnitine L-Tartrate from previous testing and I replaced the GPLC with it at a single 2 g daily dose.

"Traveling through airports with white powders may get you flagged by TSA as a potential drugs dealer!"

Steven Magee

Pandemic Supplements 3 Blood Oxygen

At the end of developing pandemic supplements 3, I did some blood oxygen readings at my home which is 600 feet above sea level in Hawaii. In March 2023 the pulse oximeter was showing:

- 93.6% average SpO2, 56.8 average BPM pulse rate: Sleeping.

- 97.5% average SpO2, 67.1 average BPM pulse rate: Sitting working on computer.

- 96.2 % average SpO2, 77.7 average BPM pulse rate: Walking around inside the home.

- 92.2% average low SpO2, 63.4 average BPM heart rate: Driving from sea level up to 6700' and back down to sea level. SpO2 started at 99% and did not fully recover when returning to sea level. It was 97% when the test finished and is consistent with the body taking about a week to recover from a short altitude test. The starting pulse rate was lower than the ending pulse rate. The test started in Keeau, passed over Highway Route 200 (Saddle Road) and finished in Kailua-Kona on Hawaii Island.

The above graphs can be seen in the following pages.

The sleep values were actually better than when I used CPAP and BiPAP sleep apnea machines in Tucson! I had not used one of these life support machines since July 2021 when I moved to near sea level in Hawaii. There was no need to. Living near to sea level cleared up my sleep apnea symptoms, which indicated it was actually central sleep apnea arising from altitude sickness from altitude hypersensitivity. Living at 2,450 feet in Tucson, Arizona, USA, appeared to have been causing altitude sickness with central sleep apnea. My altitude hypersensitivity triggers at just 1,000 feet above sea level.

In Tucson, it was normal to see SpO2 readings of 92-95% while sitting during doctors office visits. My Tucson girlfriend always tested at 98% SpO2!

"The entire time I lived at altitude in Tucson, Arizona, USA, I was never healthy."

Steven Magee

Pandemic Supplements 3 Sleeping SpO2 Graph

Blood oxygen during sleep was relatively stable and averaged 93.6% SpO2.

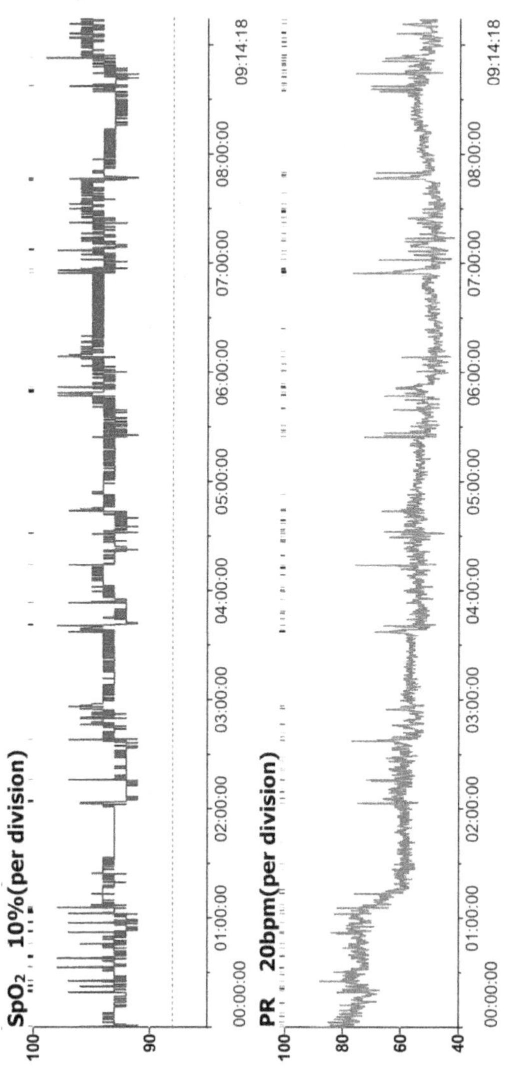

Pandemic Supplements 3 Sitting SpO2 Graph

Blood oxygen during sitting using a computer averaged 97.5% SpO2.

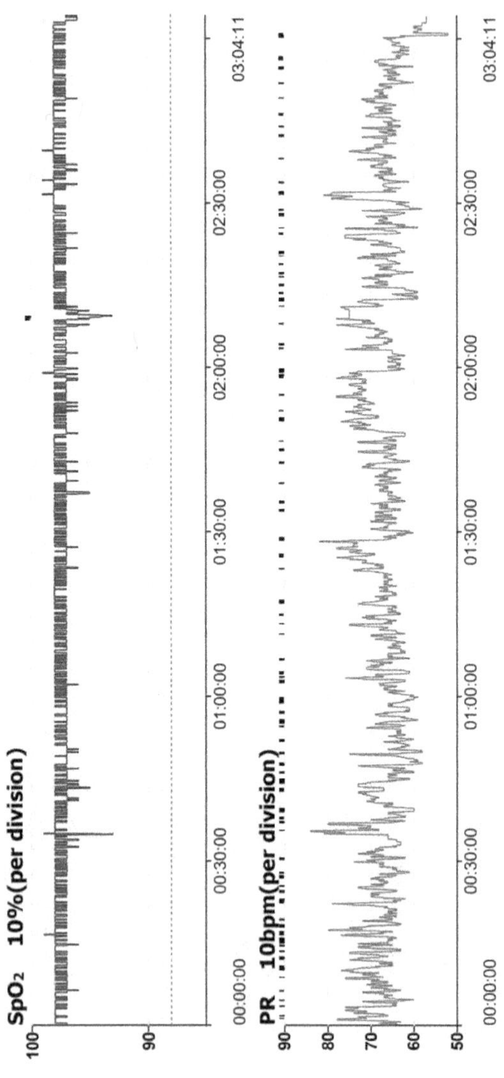

Pandemic Supplements 3 Walking SpO2 Graph

Blood oxygen during walking around inside my home averaged 96.2% SpO2.

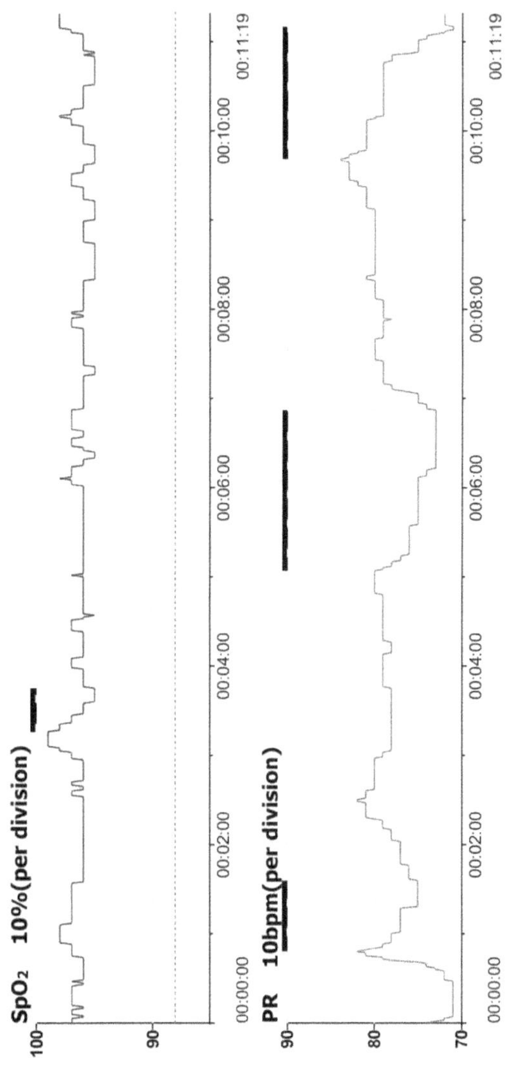

Pandemic Supplements 3 Altitude SpO2 Graph

Blood oxygen during driving up from sea level to 6,632' and back down to sea level. SpO2 low was 90% at 6,632 feet.

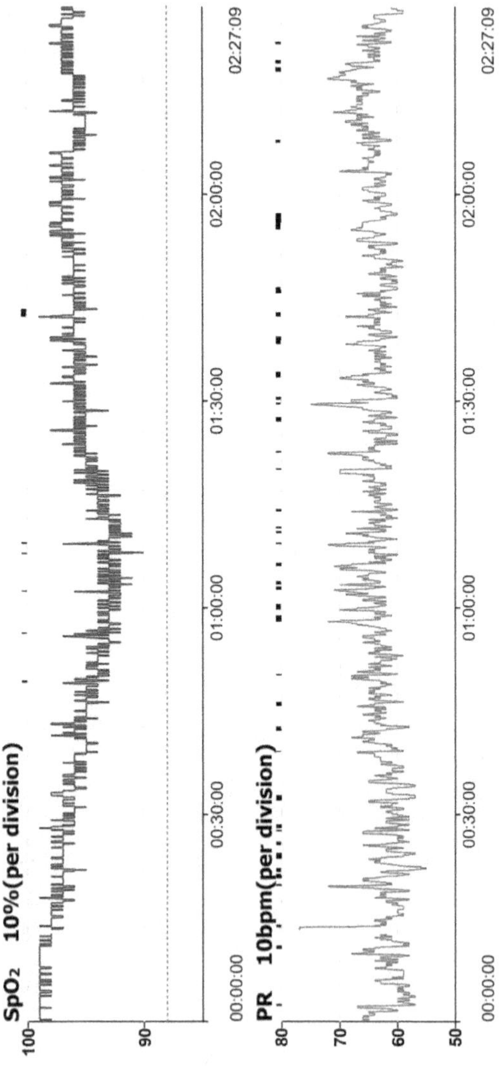

Supplement Overdose Symptoms

During developing pandemic supplements I did experience two distinct symptoms of supplement overdosing:

- Changed taste – coffee did not taste right, regardless of brand.

- Aching joints.

It is important when taking supplements to research the side effects of them to know when you may be displaying them. Changing my pandemic supplement protocol from 1 to 2 did eliminate the sore joints. My taste remained changed and I expect that will not rectify itself until I reduce my supplements to a maintenance dose of just what is essential for me.

The changed taste had coincided with a virus that I had while traveling around the USA in October and November 2022. The virus did not test positive for COVID-19, although the symptoms were similar. I had a couple of days of mild flu-like symptoms with chest pains during sleeping. It cleared up and the only symptom I was left with was all types of coffee tasting bland. It all tasted the same to me regardless of brand or roast.

"When taking nutritional supplements, it is important to know which ones have toxicity associated with them."

Steven Magee

Medical Tests

You should be aware that nutritional supplementing can affect the results of numerous medical tests. It can hide medical conditions from detection. Some of the test results known to be affected by nutritional supplements are:

- Thyroid hormone.

- Vitamin D.

- Calcium.

- Prostate specific-antigen (PSA).

- Hepatitis B.

- Hepatitis C.

- COVID-19.

- Heart attack.

- Bone density scans.

- Stool.

- Cardiac diseases.

- Endocrine disorders.

- Cancers.

- Anemias.

- Kidney disease.

- Infectious diseases.

The higher the doses of nutritional supplements are, the more likely they are to interfere with medical tests. Known supplements that cause medical test problems are:

- Riboflavin (B2).

- Biotin (B7).

- Niacin.

- Vitamin B12.

- Vitamin C.

- Vitamin E.

- Calcium.

- Iron.

- L-tryptophan.

- St. John's wort.

- 5-HTP.

Other things that are known to affect medical test results are:

- Some foods.

- Some drinks.

- Intense physical activity.

- Sunburn.

- Colds

- Infections.

- Having sex.

- Some medications or drugs.

- Lack of sleep.

- Dehydration.

You should discuss your nutritional supplement intake with your doctor prior to ordering medical tests. You should query abnormal test results that may have been adversely affected by nutritional supplements. Both "false-positive" and "false-negative" test results are known to occur.

"Nutritional supplements may give you false or inaccurate results on medical laboratory tests."

Steven Magee

Supplement Toxicity

The following supplements are well known to have the ability to cause toxicity in the human:

- An excess of vitamin B6.

- Fat soluble vitamins A, D, E, and K.

- Iron tablets.

When taking supplements and noticing the onset of unusual health issues, it is wise to review the toxicity of the supplements you are taking.

"Supplement toxicity in me was causing sore knees. I removed the suspected supplements and the sore knees disappeared!"

Steven Magee

Megacolon & Dolichocolon

Research into high altitude diseases has revealed two gastrointestinal conditions that are being seen in high altitude communities. These are:

- Megacolon: A increase in the width of the colon.

- Dolichocolon: An increase in the length of the colon with loop formation.

What does this have to do with COVID-19 and long COVID? Coronavirus can cause hypoxia to occur throughout the body. People that live in high altitude communities also have hypoxia throughout their bodies. Megacolon and dolichocolon are thought to be caused, in part, by hypoxia.

The symptoms of megacolon are:

- Constipation.

- Abdominal Pain.

- Distension and discomfort from abdominal gas.

- Obstruction.

- Fecal impaction.

- Volvulus.

- Neuropsychiatric conditions.

- Schizophrenia.

- Mental retardation.

- Central nervous system conditions.

- Cerebrovascular disease.

- Epilepsy.

Dolichocolon is believed to be a form of megacolon. The symptoms of dolichocolon are:

- Pronounced constipation.

- Meteorism.

- Indefinite colon discomfort.

- Indigestion.

- Loss of weight.

- Insomnia.

- Rumbling following the use of laxatives and cathartics, with only partial evacuation.

Megacolon and dolichocolon appear to be related to "Hirschsprung's Disease". Commonly seen in infants and children, it has the following symptoms:

- The most prominent symptom is constipation.

- Newborns:
  - Swollen belly.
  - Vomiting.
  - Constipation.
  - Gas.
  - Fussiness.
  - Diarrhea.
  - Delayed passage of meconium.

- Older children:
  - Swollen belly.
  - Chronic constipation.
  - Gas.

- ○ Failure to thrive.
- ○ Fatigue.
- Long term complications are:
  - ○ Enterocolitis.
  - ○ Megacolon.
  - ○ Bowel obstruction.
  - ○ Intestinal perforation.

I had first seen a gastroenterologist in 2006 and he had diagnosed a twist in my intestines that was causing a temporary blockage. My symptoms in 2006 were so severe I was falling over with gastrointestinal pain which would occur in the evenings after eating.

I had a colonoscopy in 2018 after a few years of my long COVID symptoms. I remember the doctor telling me afterward there were a lot of twists in my colon. I had fecal urgency at that time. The doctor found and removed a polyp in my sigmoid colon. My symptoms subsided afterwards. Based on the twists in my colon, my history of gastrointestinal problems and hypoxic exposures from a decade of working at high altitude, it seems I may have a mild version of megacolon or dolichocolon.

How does this affect nutritional absorption? Anemia and vitamin deficiencies may occur with gastrointestinal disorders. It is known to affect iron, calcium, folic acid, vitamin B12 and vitamin D specifically.

Megacolon is a known complication in COVID-19 cases.

“One of the worst health conditions I have experienced was fecal urgency!”

Steven Magee

Digestion, Fatigue & Exercise

Digestion is tied to exercise, there are no doubts about that. Sit in a chair all day long everyday and you will likely develop poor digestion. I was seeing it over and over again during researching pandemic supplements!

Sitting in a chair and using a computer all day long is a very abnormal activity for a human. Biologically, humans are hunter-gatherers and would spend their days looking for food. Food gathering is a very physical activity! Most people are burning about 2,000 calories a day with their sedentary lifestyles. The proper amount of calorie expenditure is about 4,000 calories a day for a healthy and active human.

So what happens to 2,000 calorie a day energy burning humans that are sedentary and overeating? The following conditions are typically seen:

- Obesity.

- Loss of muscle tone.

- Body profile changes and belly starts hanging out.

- Gastrointestinal issues.

- Diabetes.

- Fatigue.

- Tiredness.

- General illness.

- Diseases.

- Premature death.

What I would see when researching pandemic supplements was my digestion would degrade on the days of being sedentary on a computer. It would improve on days I was out and about and doing things. Things that would improve my digestion are:

- A day spent shopping.

- A day of gardening.

- A day of construction.

- A day out to the beach.

- A day out touring an area.

- A day of hiking.

I would never experience fatigue on these days. Two definite things would happen:

1. No fatigue on the active day.

2. Firmer stools the next day.

What is going on? This is some of what is happening:

- Increased outdoor sunlight exposure.

- Eyes are changing focus frequently.

- Increased use of muscles.

- Increased heart rate.

- Change of blood oxygenation.

- Exercise.

- Gastrointestinal tract is being massaged by movement.

- Increased calorie expenditure.

- Change of lifestyle.

- Change of brain activities.

- Talking.

By the end of researching pandemic supplements, I had become convinced that outdoor exposure in conjunction with daily movement are critical in good health. A larger daily calorie expenditure improves health. I now limit sitting at a computer to mornings only and I go outdoors and do physical work in the afternoons. It has improved my health!

I remember touring a museum that was filled with clothes from the 1800's and the guide commented that no one was fat. They had no over-sized clothes in their collection! It was before the advent of the car. Driving cars has also contributed to the sedentary lifestyle that the modern human now leads!

"The masses sitting using computers daily has coincided with a health crisis in the population."

Steven Magee

<u>Fatigue, Body Temperature & Exercise</u>

In the final stages of developing this book, I was able to go to Salem, Oregon, USA in the wintertime and test out the supplements in a cooler environment for a month. My day was spent mostly indoors at a temperature of 64 degrees Fahrenheit. 64°F was the lowest temperature on the thermostat I could tolerate while sitting working on my computer. What was noticeable was the amount of energy I had!

In Milolii, Hawaii, USA I had been taking siestas in the middle of the day when the home would get hot. I was not doing that in 64°F Oregon! It led me to conclude that keeping the body purposely cool can prevent fatigue from occurring. Allowing it to get too hot in Hawaii would cause fatigue.

Further testing in Oregon was showing that as I was going through amino acid withdrawal, I was becoming food intolerant again! The strange thing was that at 64°F I was not food intolerant. When the family I was staying with would arrive home in the evening, they would turn up the thermostat to 75°F and the home would become very warm. I was only observing food intolerance at this higher temperature. I would become very sleepy after eating the evening meal and struggle to stay awake. It would last about two hours and then slowly subside.

I had seen a similar effect in the past in Tucson, Arizona, USA. There, it was from a cool outdoor swimming pool. Every time I spent an hour in the swimming pool, I would become very energized! It did not matter how much fatigue I had at the start. Whenever I spent time in the cool outdoor swimming pool, the fatigue would disappear! It would not reappear until the next day.

In hot Hawaii, I had learned to do computer work in the cooler morning and to move outdoors and do physical work in the hotter afternoons, as my Hawaii home does not have air conditioning. The heat induced fatigue would clear through outdoor physical work.

My body eventually readjusted back to the presence of the amino acids and the food intolerance subsided again. Midday fatigue also subsided.

So what is going on? I believe it is related to the bacteria in the sedentary digestive tract. Warm up the digestive tract and bacterial overgrowth causes hyperammonemia to occur. Cool down the digestive tract and the ammonia levels of the intestinal tract reduce through reduced bacterial activity.

So why does physical activity also work to reduce fatigue? The physical activity acts like a massage on the intestinal tract and improves the digestion processes to reduce the ammonia content of the digestive tract. I have routinely noticed on days that I have a lot of physical activity, I have better stools the next day. Generally well formed and clean wiping. Physical activity from the muscles raises the ammonia levels in the blood, but not in the digestive tract.

In the swimming pool in Tucson, I was getting the benefits from both cooling and physical activity and the effect was very noticeable!

Airlines have noticed the temperature effect on the digestive tract and routinely keep their airplane high altitude cabins cool because of it. They know warmer temperatures make more people vomit!

"Food sensitivities in me are linked to hotter body temperatures."

Steven Magee

Quart Of Water

It emerged that I would feel better after eating meals if I drank a quart of water with the meal. The water appears to slow digestion and instead of the stomach being filled with a thick mash of food, it is filled with something that more resembles a fluid soup! This appears to aid digestion and keeps the body hydrated.

The water has a cooling effect on the core of the body. This cooling effect can be further enhanced if the water has ice in it. It appears beneficial in the treatment of food sensitivities if the body can be cooler than normal during and after eating.

I had noticed during many years of supplement testing that my body was more energized when on a liquid diet!

"I always drink a quart of water with every meal."

Steven Magee

Hypobaric Therapy

The three pandemic supplement protocols described were all done in conjunction with high altitude exposures. Approximately every two weeks I would drive up to 6,632 feet to see how the body was responding to the supplements at high altitude.

Supplement absorption is known to be affected by high altitude exposures and it is unclear if my recovery on the supplements is linked to these exposures causing increased absorption into the brain and the body. The brain is known to be adversely affected by high altitude exposures and the term "Summit Brain" is well known. The brain can develop "High Altitude Cerebral Edema (HACE)" causing a fluid filled brain. The lungs are also known to be strongly affected and high altitude causes a condition know as "High Altitude Pulmonary Edema (HAPE)". HAPE is very similar to the lung damage that COVID-19 causes which is fluid filled lungs. High altitude exposure is known to affect every organ in the body to some extent.

High altitude exposures also alter the body chemistry. As such, the pandemic supplements in this book have been administered in two settings:

- Near sea level at 600 feet.

- At high altitude at 6,632 feet in a hypobaric environment for the sea level adapted human.

The high altitude exposures are a form of "Hypobaric Therapy" that have been administered to the body every two weeks. While there is a page on Wikipedia that describes high pressure "Hyperbaric Therapy", there is no such page that describes the low pressure hypobaric therapy I have been using in conjunction with pandemic supplements.

Testing was indicating that increased supplement absorption was occurring and there may be a window of altitude that this occurs at. In me it appeared to be occurring in the range of 2,500 to 3,500 feet above sea level and I call this:

Altitude Nutrient Absorption Window

During the time I was developing pandemic supplements in Hawaii, I would see frequent reactions that were unique to specific altitudes. They would not be seen below the altitude nutrient absorption window and they would not be seen above it. As such, certain supplements appear to have increased absorption inside of the altitude nutrient absorption window. It is unclear if my recovery was, in part, from exposing the body regularly to high altitude and to passing through the altitude nutrient absorption window.

"I appear to be pioneering 'Hypobaric Therapy'!"

Steven Magee

Altitude Hypersensitivity Supplements At Altitude

The supplements detailed in this book to reduce altitude hypersensitivity are a treatment, not a cure. There is no known cure for altitude hypersensitivity.

My altitude hypersensitivity triggers at 1,000 feet above sea level. I was able to spend a few days living at 1,400 feet and I noticed the following:

- Sexual functioning was reduced.

- I became dizzy for several seconds after leaving a hot jacuzzi.

The next day was spent living at near sea level and no dizziness was observed when leaving the hot jacuzzi. Sexual functioning was normal.

It is important if you have altitude hypersensitivity to recognize that your body is going to behave differently at altitudes that have triggered past altitude sickness. Even when taking supplements that cause the altitude sickness symptoms to subside, you may develop health conditions at altitude.

I practice avoidance with altitudes above several hundred feet and these are things I now avoid:

- Air travel.

- Altitude airports.

- Altitude towns and cities.

- Altitude roads.

- Altitude vacations.

- Altitude jobs.

"As a person with Altitude Hypersensitivity, I spend my time at or near to sea level."

Steven Magee

Summary

So what have I learned since I have been researching pandemic supplements? The human body accumulates damage as it ages from environmental exposures, injuries and infections. Altitude sickness and coronavirus infections are very similar and can cause comparable damage throughout the body from hypoxia. It can make a person sensitized to just a small change in altitude or air pressure. Nutritional supplements can offset some of this damage by correcting malnutrition issues in the body and detoxifying toxins the damaged body is producing.

It is no secret the medical profession struggles with long COVID patients. They appear to stay sickly under their care and throwing prescription drugs and medical devices at their unusual health conditions can make them sicker! Many of my long COVID symptoms were misdiagnosed during years of visits to numerous doctors. I was never referred to a nutritionist, despite having serious food intolerance for years.

The mental health profession were very disappointing. I was surprised at how bad they were! They will diagnose you with a range of mental health conditions and start prescribing you potent brain drugs. When you tell them the brain drugs are making you sicker, they tell you to take more! The treatment was so bad from them that I had to stop using them to protect my own health and safety!

Mental illness is a common diagnosis that doctors fall back onto when they do not understand what is wrong with the patient. You need to be very careful about interacting with doctors with this diagnosis. If you start talking about poisoning with them, they may say it is your mental illness making you paranoid and you may get locked up in the mental health hospital! Be very careful about your interactions with doctors once you have a mental illness diagnosis! They have the power to institutionalize you.

I was attending an army of doctors from 2015 to 2021 with long COVID symptoms. Many were at the university research hospital. They could not accurately diagnose me. What was I telling them? The sickness I have feels like altitude sickness! I have looked up my symptoms and it matches poisoning! They could not diagnose altitude hypersensitivity and ammonia poisoning. Nothing showed up on their many medical tests to indicate these conditions were present.

My regular doctors visits extended much further back to 2006, the 2015 long COVID symptoms just added to my health issues! This is how they treated me from 2006 to 2021:

- Lung damage and asthma was treated with numerous inhalers. The actual treatment was to move to sea level.

- Sleep apnea and bruxism were treated with an anti-back device, stimulants, CPAP and BiPAP machines. The CPAP and BiPAP machines had been given to me with the pressure setting too high and were actually making me sicker! The actual treatment was to move to sea level, sleep on my front and take magnesium.

- Mental illness was treated with potent brain drugs. The actual treatment was to identify the altitude hypersensitivity and ammonia poisoning, take amino acids and move to sea level.

- Fatigue was treated with stimulants. The actual treatment was to identify protein intolerance and disrupted circadian rhythms, take amino acids, move to sea level and live in a tent outside for several months.

- Heart arrhythmia was being treated with numerous prescription medications. The actual treatment was nutritional support for the heart and to move to sea level.

- Gastrointestinal problems were treated with a colonoscopy and removal of a polyp. They got part of the treatment right. The full treatment was live culture support from yogurt, nutritional support, daily exercise, a cooler environment and move to sea level.

- Fungal toenails were treated by removing the toenails and painting an anti-fungal onto the new nails which did not work. The correct treatment appears to be an oral anti-fungal for several months, painting an anti-fungal onto the toenails, treating the ammonia poisoning and move to sea level.

- Food intolerance was never treated. The correct treatment was to adopt a comprehensive nutritional support system that included amino acids, a low protein diet and move to sea level.

- Altitude sickness was never treated. The correct treatment was to move to sea level and take L-Carnitine and glycine.

- Poisoning was never treated. The correct treatment was lysine, carnitine and arginine nutritional supplementation, detoxify from heavy metals poisoning and move to sea level.

My treatment from the doctors ranged from almost nothing through to lots of prescription drugs. The treatment varied between each doctor. Some were watching how my health was degrading and monitoring it, while others were trying to use prescription drugs to fix it. I had one doctor that was trying to tell me it was "All in my mind!". I left that doctor after hearing that.

Be aware the modern medical profession has no real incentive to fix you. Financially, the doctor is in a much better position if you stay sick, because you will be a regular at the office and will be producing a nice income for the doctor!

There are no doubts that the modern medical system is under the influence of pharmaceutical companies. Many of their expensive drugs work no better than nutritional supplements! But the prescriptions may come with nasty side effects. Some of my prescription medications were $500 per month for each medicine!

By the time I was done with the medical profession in 2021, I had been under the care of numerous primary care doctors, I had been under the care of numerous specialist doctors and I had been attending the four main hospitals in Tucson including the university research hospital.

At the age of fifty-three I will never be cured of permanent biological damage. I was fortunate I had some lucky breaks that improved my mental functioning to the point I could correctly self diagnose my symptoms. One of these was my ex-girlfriend switching out my diet to a gluten free one. Had this not happened, I would still be misdiagnosed!

I call my disease "Magee's Disease", as I have not been able to find a medical condition in the published medical literature that covers the full range of health issues I had. As such, I believe Magee's disease is a new and previously undocumented health condition in the general population. This explains why all of the numerous doctors I saw were unable to make a diagnosis of Magee's disease and prescribe the correct treatment.

My recovery has been so successful that I have not been to a doctors office since I left Arizona in July 2021. I have medical insurance in Hawaii and I have never needed to use it in almost two years. I do not have a primary care doctor. At the peak of the sickness in Tucson, I was averaging a doctors visit every few weeks! I was under the care of a wide range of specialist doctors at the time.

My other books provide further information on health and you may want to consider reading them:

- Magee's Disease.

- Curing Electromagnetic Hypersensitivity.

- Toxic Altitude.

- Toxic Electricity.

- Toxic Health.

- Toxic Light.

- Solar Radiation, Global Warming, and Human Disease.

I hope you enjoyed this book and I wish you the very best of health.

"I was surprised the USA medical profession could not diagnose low blood oxygen levels, sensitivity to abnormal air, food intolerance, malnutrition, a urea cycle disorder, altitude hypersensitivity, loss of circadian rhythm and loss of moonlight synchronization."

Steven Magee

<u>References</u>

Books:

- Brain Longevity by Dharma Singh Khalsa.

- Brain Maker: The Power of Gut Microbes to Heal and Protect Your Brain - for Life by David Perlmutter with Kristin Loberg.

- HEAVY METALS DETOX: The fast-track to a healthier version of YOU! by James Lilley.

- No Grain, No Pain: A 30-Day Diet for Eliminating the Root Cause of Chronic Pain by Peter Osborne.

- Prescription For Nutritional Healing by James F. Balch, MD & Phyllis A Balch, CNC.

- The Complete Low-FODMAP Diet: A Revolutionary Plan for Managing IBS and Other Digestive Disorders by Sue Shepherd.

- The Plant Paradox - The Hidden Dangers in "Healthy" Foods That Cause Disease and Weight Gain by Dr. Steven R Gundry MD.

- Wheat Belly by William Davis.

Internet:

- Dietary supplement:
  - https://en.wikipedia.org/wiki/Dietary_supplement

- Linus Pauling Institute's Micronutrient Information Center:
  - https://lpi.oregonstate.edu/mic/

- NIH Dietary Supplement Fact Sheets:

- ○ https://ods.od.nih.gov/factsheets/list-all/
- Mayo Clinic nutrition and healthy eating:
  - ○ https://www.mayoclinic.org/healthy-lifestyle/nutrition-and-healthy-eating/basics/nutrition-basics/hlv-20049477
- The Nutrition Source at Harvard College:
  - ○ https://www.hsph.harvard.edu/nutritionsource/
- WebMD Vitamins & Supplements:
  - ○ https://www.webmd.com/vitamins/index

"I found my correct diagnosis in books and on the internet."

Steven Magee

Most At Risk Of Hypoxia

The most at risk of hypoxia illnesses and diseases are:

- Space.
  - Astronauts.
  - Tourists.
- Aviation workers.
  - Pilots.
  - Airline cabin crew.
  - Frequent fliers.
- High altitude astronomy workers.
- Winter sports.
  - Skiers.
  - Snowboarders.
- Mountain hikers.
- High altitude hikers.
- Mountain workers.
  - Lodges.
  - Resorts.
  - Some national parks.
- Forest workers.
- People that live in altitude cities.
- Drivers and truckers.
- Radio and television transmitter workers.
- Cell phone tower workers.

- People with pre-existing health conditions.

- People with sea level adapted genetics.

- People with a hole in the heart (ASD).

- People that have breathed industrial gasses.

- People that have breathed medical gasses.

- People that live inside poorly ventilated homes with gas appliances.

- People that have been exposed to hypoxic environments.

- People that have had a coronavirus infection.

- People with Long COVID.

"Truckers that drive all over the USA are often in hypoxic environments!"

Steven Magee

<u>Acknowledgments</u>

This book was influenced by:

- Those that are developing the important science of environmental health and bringing it to the masses.

- My family for providing support during my prolonged and mysterious illness.

"Mysterious disabling illnesses will make you dependent on people."

Steven Magee

About The Author

About Steven Magee CEng MIET BEng Hons, member of Environmental Radiation LLC:

Steven was born in the United Kingdom (UK) and started his career at one of the largest university research and teaching hospitals in Europe. Working in the electrical engineering group, he obtained a Bachelors with Honors in Electrical and Electronic Engineering. Human health was a strong draw and he moved into the biomedical team, serving the regions hospitals. During this time he developed a fascination for human illness and disease and the causes of it, many of which were not understood.

He joined the Isaac Newton Group of Telescopes in 1999 and went to live in La Palma. La Palma is part of the Canary Islands, governed by Spain. During this time he worked with the leading European astronomers and developed his astronomical and optics skills. He became fluent in Spanish and their culture.

In 2001 he became a Chartered Electrical Engineer and joined the W. M. Keck Observatory in Hawaii. This was the world's leading astronomical facility and home to the world's two largest segmented mirror telescopes. Steven developed segmented optics and interferometry skills while working alongside world leading astronomers. He was the assistant to Nobel Prize winners including the fourth woman to win the prize in physics, Andrea Ghez. During this time Steven constructed his own off-grid solar powered home in the last of the traditional Hawaiian fishing villages in Miloli'i, Hawaii. He learned Hawaiian Pidgin English and the Hawaiian culture during his time there.

In 2006, Steven became the Director of the MDM Observatory in Sells, Arizona, USA. Working for Columbia University and later, Dartmouth College, he developed the facility to modern standards. He learned an appreciation of the Native Americans and their culture from the Tohono O'odham Nation.

In 2008, Steven joined the solar power revolution that was sweeping the USA and commissioned the largest CIGS thin film solar photovoltaic installation in the world.

A year later he became the Florida Power and Light (FPL) Manager of the DeSoto Next Generation Solar Energy Center, which was the largest solar photovoltaic utility power generation plant ever built in the USA. The system rated power was quoted as 25,000,000 watts AC with over 90,500 solar modules that were mounted to 158 single-axis tracker systems in three hundred acres of land and it was opened by President Obama.

He went on to develop the solar photovoltaic team for a large international company.

In 2010 he started to research radiation and publish the leading books on the subject.

He became a USA citizen in 2017 and continues to be interested in global radiation health effects and how it impacts over seven billion people on planet Earth.

"I had a very interesting career that sent me into ill health and onto disability."

Steven Magee

Author Contact

This is the Environmental Radiation LLC website:

- www.environmentalradiation.com

You can follow the Twitter feed at:

- Steven Magee @EnvironmentEMR
- https://twitter.com/EnvironmentEMR

The Facebook page is:

- https://www.facebook.com/EnvironmentEMR

You may find my other books useful:

Architecture

- **Solar Reflections for Architects, Engineers, and Human Health**: This book is a comprehensive collection of images, diagrams, and notes that document the effects of sunlight in architecture. This is essential information for architects, engineers, and the medical profession. The discovery of the "Multiple-Sun" effect in architecture is detailed and this book is illustrated in color.

Climate Change

- **Solar Radiation, Global Warming, and Human Disease**: This book examines the modern development of the Earth and the potential impacts on global warming and human disease. The destruction of the forests for modern agricultural use appears to have effects that are not fully understood and these are explored. Radiation deficiency and radiation overloading are investigated to see if they are factors in many illnesses and diseases.

Human Health

- **Hypoxia, Mental Illness & Chronic Fatigue**: This book examines the many aspects of hypoxia that may lead to the development of mental illness and chronic fatigue. Modern society is filled with hypoxia experiences that are well known for their ability to affect brain functioning and energy levels.   Solutions are explored for underlying conditions that doctors may have missed.

- **Magee's Disease**: Magee's Disease, Summit Brain, Altitude Sickness, COVID-19 and Long COVID are all related. This book delves into the silent world of hypoxia and what it can do to people. The failings of the modern medical profession are examined and solutions to the hypoxic Magee's Disease are explored.

- **Night Shift Recovery:** Unusual work shifts may lead to the development of Shift Work Disorder. Shift work is well known for its ability to degrade human health. Recovery can be achieved and solutions are explored for underlying conditions that doctors may have missed.

- **Solar Radiation – A Cause of Illness and Cancer?** Illness and cancers have become part of our modern culture. It has been discovered that extremely high levels of man-made solar radiation exist in modern society. Could this be the one of the causes of illness and cancers? This book examines the increase in solar radiation and applies it to human health.

- **Summit Brain:** Summit Brain is a term used to describe the health issues that appear in people that commute to very high altitude. This book explores the biological reasons that cause Summit Brain to occur. Recovery from Summit Brain can be achieved and solutions are explored for underlying conditions that doctors may have missed.

Nutrition

- **Pandemic Supplements:** Steven Magee became disabled by a mystery flu-like sickness he caught from an international university professor. During the COVID-19 pandemic, he realized his mysterious range of symptoms matched a new sickness called Long COVID. This book explores the nutritional supplements he used to recover his mental and physical health.

Toxicity

- **Toxic Altitude:** Toxic Altitude explores the biological reasons that cause Altitude Sickness to occur in sea level adapted humans. Recovery from the long term effects of Altitude Sickness can be achieved and solutions are explored for underlying conditions that doctors may have missed.

- **Toxic Electricity:** Random aches and pains? Fatigue? Insomnia? Facial pains? Irregular heartbeats? Sick kids? Relationship problems? Blotchy skin? Anxiety? Toxic electricity takes a look at the electrical system and asks the question: Is this one of the most toxic endeavors that humanity has ever engaged in?

- **Toxic Health:** Toxic Health takes a look at the pollution that may be in your local environment and relates it to the health problems that it can cause. Pollution in the human environment is only just starting to be understood and something as innocent as light may be able to make you really ill! There are many examples of commonplace items in your environment that may have the ability to affect your health. In particular, we will investigate if modern city life is the most toxic thing of all to the modern human!

- **Toxic Light:** Toxic Light takes a look at the light pollution that may be in your local environment and relates it to the health problems that it may cause. Light in the human environment is only just starting to be understood and something as innocent as your sunglasses may be able to make you ill! There are many examples of commonplace items in your environment that may have the ability to affect your health. Get ready for enlightenment about the most important human nutrient of light!

Forensics

- **Electrical Forensics:** Electrical Forensics examines the many aspects of electricity, electronics and wireless communications that may lead to unusual behaviors to occur in humans. Electromagnetic interference is well known for its ability to affect mental functioning and human health. Electrical Forensics demonstrates how to identify toxic electromagnetic environments that may be the root cause of accidents and crimes.

- **Health Forensics:** Health Forensics examines the many aspects of modern society that may lead to unusual behaviors to occur in humans. Modern society has adopted habits that are well known for their ability to affect mental functioning and human health. Health Forensics demonstrates how to identify toxic human environments that may be the root cause of accidents and crimes.

- **Light Forensics**: Light Forensics examines the many aspects of modern lighting that may lead to unusual behaviors to occur in humans. Modern society has adopted optical products that are well known for their ability to affect mental functioning and human health. Light Forensics demonstrates how to identify toxic light that may be the root cause of accidents and crimes.

Religion

- **Solar Radiation, the Book of Revelations, and the Era of Light – Part 1:** Welcome to the Era of Light! Light has long been known to be essential nourishment for the human body. We will explore the different types of light that are present on Earth and relate it to human health and nature. Light is discussed extensively in the Bible and we will see if we can associate our findings to it. Finally, we will investigate if the Industrial Revolution has created the ultimate toxin of poisonous sunlight!

Professional

- **Engineering Science and Education Journal Volume: 11, Issue: 4, Active Control Systems for Large Segmented Optical Mirrors:** A new generation of optical telescopes is on the drawing board. These will be true giants with primary mirrors having a diameter of up to 100 meters. The technology that will enable this revolution to take place was developed at the W. M. Keck Observatory in Hawaii, where the world's largest segmented mirrors are in daily use. This article looks at how the W. M. Keck Observatory proved the mirror technology that will be behind this new generation of telescopes.

Solar Photovoltaic

- **Complete Solar Photovoltaics for Residential, Commercial, and Utility Systems:** Steven Magee has combined his three top selling books on solar power systems into one edition. Complete Solar Photovoltaics will train you on solar photovoltaics and show you how to design grid connected solar photovoltaic power systems. Operations and maintenance is detailed to enable you to have a complete understanding of solar photovoltaics from start to finish.

- **Solar Photovoltaics for Consumers, Utilities, and Investors:** This book details solar photovoltaic systems for consumers, utilities and investors. This would encompass residential, commercial and utility systems that are connected to the utility grid. There is a discussion of the different technologies available for the consumer and their advantages and disadvantages. For the utilities, there is invaluable advice on planning and constructing large projects. For the investor, forward looking statements try to predict the future of solar photovoltaics.

- **Solar Photovoltaic Training for Residential, Commercial, and Utility Systems:** This book details solar photovoltaic training for those who are interested in this area and also for those who are already working in the field. This would encompass residential, commercial, and utility systems that are connected to the utility grid. It is a comprehensive overview of a rapidly growing world of solar photovoltaic power generation technology.

- **Solar Photovoltaic Design for Residential, Commercial, and Utility Systems:** This book details how to design reliable solar photovoltaic power generation systems from a residential system, progressing to a commercial system, and finishing at the largest utility power generation systems. By following the guidelines in this book and your local solar photovoltaic electrical codes, you will be able to design trouble free solar power systems that give many years of reliable operation. When designed well, solar photovoltaic power generation is an excellent source of electrical power that results in much lower electricity bills, the power company will even refund you for the excess energy generated by your system if it is large enough. Building a grid tied solar power system is a relatively easy task. Given the large amount of government and electrical utility financial incentives that are available, it is a great time to join in the solar power revolution that is taking place in the world today.

- **Solar Photovoltaic Operation and Maintenance for Residential, Commercial, and Utility Systems:** This book details how to operate and maintain residential, commercial, and utility solar photovoltaic systems that are connected to the utility grid. By following the guidelines in this book you will be able to operate and maintain solar power systems that should give many years of reliable operation. Invaluable trouble shooting advice will aid in returning your system to full operation in the event of a problem.

- **Solar Photovoltaic DC Calculations for Residential, Commercial, and Utility Systems:** This book details how to run calculations for the DC circuit of solar photovoltaic systems. This would encompass residential, commercial, and utility systems that are connected to the utility grid. It covers the range of conditions that solar photovoltaic modules are exposed to throughout the year and shows how to incorporate these into an effective DC circuit that is well designed and reliable.

- **Solar Photovoltaic Resource for Residential, Commercial, and Utility Systems:** This book is a resource of information that is used in the solar photovoltaic field. This would encompass residential, commercial, and utility systems that are connected to the utility grid. It is a comprehensive collection of notes, diagrams, pictures and charts for a rapidly growing world of solar photovoltaic power generation technology. This book is illustrated in color.

Solar Radiation

- **Solar Irradiance and Insolation for Power Systems:** This book is a resource of information that is used in the solar power generation field. This would encompass residential, commercial, and utility systems that are connected to the utility grid. It is a comprehensive collection of notes, diagrams, pictures, and charts for a rapidly growing world of solar photovoltaic power generation technology. This book is illustrated in color.

- **Solar Site Selection for Power Systems:** This book is a comprehensive collection of images, diagrams, and notes that document the effects of light and heat in the solar power generation field. This would encompass residential, commercial, and utility systems that are connected to the utility grid. This is essential information for a rapidly growing world of solar power generation technology. This book is illustrated in color.

You can search "Steven Magee Books" for the very latest publications.

www.youtube.com videos supporting the ideas in the books can be found by searching StevenMageeBooks:

- https://www.youtube.com/user/StevenMageeBooks

"Writing books is by far the most interesting thing I have done in life."

Steven Magee

Book Reviews

Complete Solar Photovoltaics for Residential, Commercial, and Utility Systems rated 5 out of 5 stars.

Reviewed by Amanda Bassett on December 4, 2015 titled "Perfect read".

Perfect for solar farm studies. Takes the reader from basics who doesn't know a sausage about electricity to turning it into a business. We are considering doing just this in Arizona ourselves.

Curing Electromagnetic Hypersensitivity rated 5 out of 5 stars.

Reviewed by Ann on on January 31, 2015 titled "Don't miss the message here folks!".

This book says a lot abut the importance of not only avoiding radiation but the necessity of taking steps to replenish and rebalance the body's own electrical system in order to build resistance to the unavoidable radiation exposures that we live with in this world. I have suffered with EHS and MCS and over the years I have gotten the most improvement by tracking my nutrient/mineral levels and supplementing accordingly. I am not surprised that the author has gotten his health back by "charging his battery, " so to speak. I have always believed that the most effective way to prevent or cure disease is to improve the "terrain" of the body. Thanks to the author for pointing this out and sharing the specifics!

Electrical Forensics rated 5 out of 5 stars.

Review by John Puccetti on October 27, 2013 titled "Dangers of electricity"

Steven has made many of the health problems of our century known in his book. But what will we do is this information? We live in a corporate dictatorship that masquerades as democracy.

Health Forensics rated 5 out of 5 stars.

Reviewed by honesT on July 26, 2014 titled "Incredible insights you would have never thought of :O".

Incredible insights, seriously Steve nails it again. If your just an average person looking for some insight about the whole EMF thing this is for you 100%. If your a seasoned EMF pro looking for some new insights this book is worth it`s weight in gold and you will, I have no doubt in my mind take in new knowledge that will no doubt open doors. You do not have to read this book from cover to cover, just pick any chapter read and be amazed what you learn. So many areas are covered in this book, it`s really like a mini encyclopedia for EMF and how that`s affecting our surroundings that in turn affect our body, mind and emotions. I really can`t say enough I mean just look at the price it`s practically free :]

Solar Photovoltaic Training for Residential, Commercial and Utility Systems rated 5 out of 5 stars.

Reviewed by Kyle William Loshure on November 13, 2016 titled "Solar power is #1"

Thank you for your work!

Solar Radiation, Global Warming and Human Disease rated 5 out of 5 stars.

Reviewed by Donato Cobarrubias on October 4, 2014 titled "Five Stars"

Great book and great info! I learned a lot!

Toxic Electricity rated 5 out of 5 stars.

Review by Sam Wieder on December 13, 2013 titled "A Most Illuminating, Educational, and Helpful Book"

Toxic Electricity provides a clear and comprehensive description of the many ways in which electrical fields impact human health and offers simple steps that anyone can take to live a more vibrant life in our electrically toxic world. The author does a masterful job of presenting some fairly complex concepts in a way that is easily understandable. Reading this book will give you a deeper understanding of how unseen radiation in your living and working environment may be impacting you. If you've been battling different health challenges or are chronically tired for no apparent reason, this book may very well open your eyes to some answers that will help you regain your health and your life.

Toxic Light rated 5 out of 5 stars.

Titled "Five Stars".

Reviewed by Amazon Customer on September 17, 2018

Great book, lots of information about light you never hear about anywhere.

"When I saw the five star reviews appearing, I knew the research was progressing in the right direction."

Steven Magee

www.ingramcontent.com/pod-product-compliance
Lightning Source LLC
Chambersburg PA
CBHW070826250726
48662CB00003B/1102